LIPPINCOTT'S REVIEW SERIES

Mental Health and Psychiatric Nursing

LIPPINCOTT'S REVIEW SERIES

Mental Health and Psychiatric Nursing

J.B. LIPPINCOTT COMPANY
Philadelphia

New York • London • Hagerstown

Sponsoring Editor: **Donna L. Hilton, RN, BSN**
Coordinating Editorial Assistant: **Susan Perry**
Project Editor: **Melissa McGrath**
Indexer: **Alexandra Nickerson**
Designer: **Doug Smock**
Production Manager: **Helen Ewan**
Production Coordinator: **Maura Murphy**
Compositor: **Pine Tree Composition, Inc.**
Printer/Binder: **R. R. Donnelley & Sons Company**
Cover Printer: **The Lehigh Press, Inc.**

6 5 4 3 2

Library of Congress Cataloging-in-Publication Data

Lippincott's review series : mental health and psychiatric nursing.
    p.   cm.
  Includes bibliographical references and index.
  ISBN 0-397-54773-0
  1. Psychiatric nursing. I. J. B. Lippincott Company. II. Title:
Mental health and psychiatric nursing.
  [DNLM: 1. Mental Health—examination questions. 2. Psychiatric
Nursing—examination questions. WY 18 L7651]
RC440.L57 1992
610.73'68'076—dc20
DNLM/DLC
for Library of Congress   91-29908
                                       CIP

CONTRIBUTING AUTHORS

Nu-Vision, Inc.
Paula S. Cokingtin, RN, EdD, President
Kathy D. Robinson, RN, MSN, Vice President
Carolyn H. Brose, RN, EdD, Vice President
Linda N. Kohlman, RN, MN, Associate

Elaine Darst, RN, PhD

Assistant Professor
Research College of Nursing
Kansas City, Missouri

Barbara Dancy, RN, PhD

Assistant Professor
University of Illinois at Chicago
College of Nursing
Chicago, Illinois

Laina M. Gerace, RN, PhD

Assistant Professor
University of Illinois at Chicago
College of Nursing
Chicago, Illinois

Carla A. Lee, RN, C, PhD, FAAN

Assistant Professor
Wichita State University
Wichita, Kansas

Ann Milius, RN, MA, CS

Clinical Specialist, Section Nurse
The Meninger Clinic
Topeka, Kansas

Barbara A. Zeugner, RN, MS

Instructor
Louisiana State University
New Orleans, Louisiana

REVIEWERS

Carol J. Bininger, RN, PhD

Assistant Professor
Ohio State University
College of Nursing
Columbus, Ohio

Kathleen Blanchfield, RN, MS

Human Resources Department
Evangel Health Services
Oakbrook, Illinois

Frederick Bozett, RN, DNS

Professor
University of Oklahoma
Health Sciences Center
Oklahoma City, Oklahoma

Robert Kus, RN, PhD

Associate Professor
University of Iowa
Iowa City, Iowa

Joan Fopma-Loy, RN, MSN

Assistant Professor of Nursing
Indiana University East
Richmond, Indiana

Sue Schuler, RN, PhD

Director of Nursing
Milwaukee County Mental Health Complex
Milwaukee, Wisconsin

INTRODUCTION

Lippincott's Review Series is designed to help you in your study of the key subject areas in nursing. The series consists of four books, one in each core nursing subject area:

Medical-Surgical Nursing
Pediatric Nursing
Maternal-Newborn Nursing
Mental Health and Psychiatric Nursing

Each book contains a comprehensive outline content review, chapter study questions and answer keys with rationales for correct and incorrect responses, and a comprehensive examination and answer key with rationales for correct and incorrect responses.

Lippincott's Review Series was planned and developed in response to your requests for outline review books that address each major subject area and also contain a self-test mechanism. These books meet the need for comprehensive subject review books that will also assist you in identifying your strong and weak areas of knowledge. Each book is a complete source for review and self-assessment of a single core subject—all four together provide an excellent comprehensive review of entry-level nursing.

Each book is all-inclusive of the content addressed in major textbooks. The content outline review uses a consistent nursing process format throughout and addresses nursing care for well and ill clients. Also included are such necessary additional topics as developmental and life-cycle issues, health assessment, patient teaching, and other concepts including growth and development, nutrition, pharmacology, and anatomy, physiology, and pathophysiology.

You can use the books in this series in several different ways. Overall, you can use them as subject reviews to augment general study throughout your basic nursing program and as a review to prepare for the National Council Licensure Examination (NCLEX-RN). How you use each book depends on your individual needs and preferences and on whether you review each chapter systematically or concentrate only on those chapters whose subject areas are particularly problematic or challenging. You may instead choose to use the comprehensive examination as a self-assessment opportunity to evaluate your knowledge base before you review the content outline. Likewise, you can use the study questions for pre- or post-testing after study, followed by the comprehensive examination as a means of evaluating your knowledge and competencies of an entire subject area.

Regardless of how you use the books, one of the strengths of the series is the self-assessment opportunity it offers in addition to guidance in studying and reviewing content. The chapter study questions and comprehensive examination questions have been carefully developed to cover all topics in the outline review. Most importantly, each question is categorized according to the components of the National Council of State Boards of Nursing Licensing Examination (NCLEX).

- Cognitive Level: Knowledge, Comprehension, Application, or Analysis
- Client Need: Safe, Effective Care Environment (Safe Care); Physiological Integrity (Physiologic); Psychosocial Integrity (Psychosocial); and Health Promotion and Maintenance (Health Promotion)
- Phase of the Nursing Process: Assessment, Analysis (Dx), Planning, Implementation, Evaluation

For those questions not related to a client need or to a phase of the nursing process, NA (not applicable) will be used, as in questions that test knowledge of a basic science.

Unlike the NCLEX examination that tests the cumulative knowledge needed for safe practice by an entry-level nurse, these practice tests systematically evaluate the knowledge base that serves as the building block for the entire nursing educational process. In this way, you can prepare for the NCLEX examination throughout your course of study. Good study habits throughout your educational program are not only the best way to ensure on-going success, but also will prove the most beneficial way to prepare for the licensing examination.

Keep in mind that these books are not intended to replace formal learning. They cannot substitute for textbook reading, discussion with instructors, or class attendance. Every effort has been made to provide accurate and current information, but class attendance and interaction with an instructor will provide invaluable information not found in books. Used correctly, these books will help you increase understanding, improve comprehension, evaluate strengths and weaknesses in areas of knowledge, increase productive study time, and as a result help you improve your grades.

MONEY BACK GUARANTEE—Lippincott's Review Series will help you study more effectively during coursework throughout your educational program and help you prepare for quizzes and tests, including the NCLEX exam. If you buy and use any of the four volumes in Lippincott's Review Series and fail the NCLEX exam, simply send us verification of your exam results and your copy of the review book to the address below. We will promptly send you a check for our suggested list price.

Lippincott's Review Series
J. B. Lippincott Company
227 East Washington Square
Philadelphia, PA 19106-3780

CONTENTS

LIPPINCOTT'S REVIEW SERIES

Mental Health and Psychiatric Nursing

Professional Role
and Practice
of Mental Health
and Psychiatric Nursing

I. Overview
A. Evolution of mental health and psychiatric nursing

1. Among her many accomplishments, Florence Nightingale (1850s) noted that patient care must involve psychologic and social, as well as physiologic, aspects.
2. In the 1880s, Linda Richards promoted better care for psychiatric

patients and directed the first school for mental health and psychiatric nursing.

3. Working as Assistant Superintendent of Nurses at the psychiatric clinic of Johns Hopkins Hospital, Harriet Baily wrote the first psychiatric nursing textbook, *Nursing Mental Diseases,* in 1920.

4. In 1937, the National League for Nursing (NLN) recommended that mental health and psychiatric nursing be included in nursing school curricula. The NLN also assumed responsibility for standardization and accreditation of psychiatric nursing education.

5. In 1948, Esther Lucille Brown wrote a report, "Nursing for the Future," recommending that psychiatric nursing schools be incorporated into the basic schools of nursing.

6. Hildegard Peplau's 1958 book *Interpersonal Relations in Nursing* presented the first major framework for psychiatric nursing practice and also emphasized the interpersonal nature of nursing and the use of psychodynamic principles in nursing practice.

7. In 1958, the American Nurses Association (ANA) established the Conference Group on Psychiatric Nursing, now known as the Council on Psychiatric and Mental Health Nursing Practice.

8. In 1973, the ANA published the first standards of mental health and psychiatric nursing practice; these standards were revised in 1982.

B. **Roles and functions of the mental health and psychiatric nurse**

1. The mental health and psychiatric nurse provides direct care to patients with mental or emotional disorders, including:
   a. Promoting self-care and independence
   b. Assisting with problem solving to facilitate activities of daily living
   c. Aiding communication and interpersonal relations
   d. Helping the patient examine behaviors and test alternatives
   e. Teaching about the disorder
   f. Administering prescribed medications and treatments

2. The nurse also is responsible for constructing and maintaining a therapeutic environment.

3. Another important nursing function involves patient and family teaching.

4. In many cases, the mental health and psychiatric nurse coordinates diverse aspects of care.

5. Acting as an advocate on behalf of the patient and family, the nurse:
   a. Teaches about rights and responsibilities
   b. Shares information about self-help groups

6. Responsibilities associated with primary prevention include:
   a. Teaching principles of mental health
   b. Teaching how to recognize and reduce stress
   c. Promoting effective family functioning

       d.   Participating in community activities related to mental health promotion

C. **Practice settings**
1. Acute care inpatient settings
   a. General community hospitals
   b. Medical centers
   c. State facilities
   d. Veterans' facilities
2. Crisis care settings
   a. Walk-in clinics
   b. Outpatient services
   c. Crisis hot line units
3. Community mental health centers
4. Private organizations
5. Ongoing care for patients with chronic mental illness
   a. Halfway houses
   b. Clinics
   c. Structured work programs and sheltered workshops
6. Partial hospitalization programs
7. Prisons

D. **Levels of care**
1. Primary prevention involves altering causative or risk factors to hinder the development of illness, and encompasses:
   a. Client and family teaching
   b. Stress reduction
   c. Psychosocial support
2. Secondary prevention focuses on reducing or minimizing the effects of mental illness; aspects include:
   a. Screening
   b. Crisis intervention
   c. Suicide prevention
   d. Short-term counseling
   e. Emergency nursing care and short-term hospitalization
3. Tertiary prevention involves minimizing long-term residual effects of illness; examples include:
   a. Rehabilitation programs
   b. Vocational training
   c. Aftercare support
   d. Partial hospitalization options

E. **Levels of practice (recognized by the ANA)**
1. Mental health and psychiatric nurse generalists
   a. Education: baccalaureate degree in nursing
   b. Practice: staff nurse in inpatient and community settings
2. Mental health and psychiatric nurse specialists
   a. Education: graduate degree in mental health and psychiatric nursing

        b.   Practice: clinical specialist and supervisory roles in inpatient and community settings

F. **Standards of practice**

    1.   The first widely accepted standards of practice were developed by the ANA's Council on Psychiatric and Mental Health Nursing Practice in 1973 and were revised in 1982.

    2.   These standards address the following:

        a.   Use of theory to guide practice

        b.   The nursing process: assessment, nursing diagnosis, planning, implementation, evaluation

        c.   Peer review for quality assurance

        d.   Continuing education

        e.   Interdisciplinary collaboration

        f.   Utilization of community health systems

        g.   Nursing research

II. Therapeutic nurse–patient relationships

A. **Elements of a therapeutic relationship**

    1.   Goal-directed and purposeful interaction involves:

        a.   Establishing a contract for the time, place, and focus of nurse–patient meetings

        b.   Planning conditions for termination at the onset of and throughout the relationship

    2.   Roles and responsibilities should be clearly defined; the nurse is the professional helper and facilitator, and the patient's needs and problems are the focus of the relationship.

    3.   Confidentiality is maintained by:

        a.   Sharing information only with professional staff

        b.   Apprising the patient of all information to be shared beforehand

        c.   Obtaining the patient's permission to share information with any others outside of the health care team

    4.   Therapeutic behaviors by the nurse include:

        a.   Self-awareness of thoughts, feelings, behaviors

        b.   Clarification of personal values

        c.   Ability to listen accurately and empathically

        d.   Ability to communicate effectively

        e.   Ability to set realistic goals

        f.   Ability to work collaboratively with the patient

        g.   Good sense of ethics and responsibility

B. **Phases of a therapeutic relationship**

    1.   The *orientation (assessment and analysis) phase* involves:

        a.   Developing trust and open communication

        b.   Assessing the patient's reason for seeking help or hospitalization

        c.   Establishing mutually agreed-upon goals

        d.   Developing a therapeutic contract (see Display 1–1)

        e.   Formulating nursing diagnoses

  2. In the *working (planning and implementation) phase:*

        a.   Interventions are planned to meet patient goals.

        b.   Expression of thoughts and feelings is facilitated.

        c.   Problems are explored.

        d.   Constructive coping mechanisms are encouraged.

        e.   Alternative, more adaptive behaviors are practiced and evaluated.

        f.   Resistances and testing behavior are worked through.

  3. The *termination (evaluation) phase* involves:

        a.   Evaluating therapeutic outcomes

        b.   Expressing feelings about termination

        c.   Observing for regressive behavior

        d.   Evaluating the nurse–patient relationship

C. **Therapeutic communication (or facilitative communication)**

  1. Structural elements of communication include:

        a.   Sender: originator of the message

        b.   Message: information transmitted

        c.   Receiver: recipient of the message

        d.   Feedback: response of the receiver to the message

        e.   Context: setting in which communication takes place

  2. Nonverbal communication techniques include:

        a.   Kinetics: body movements such as gestures, facial expressions, and other mannerisms

        b.   Proxemics, the space between communicators (e.g., intimate space, up to 18 inches; personal space, 18 inches to 4 ft; social-consultative space, 9 to 12 ft; and public space, more than 12 ft apart)

        c.   Touch

        d.   Silence

  3. Variables influencing communication include:

        a.   Perception: one's viewpoint about the situation

        b.   Values: one's beliefs about what is desirable

DISPLAY 1–1.
Essential Elements of a Nurse–Patient Contract

Nurse and patient know each other's names.

Patient understands the nurse's role.

Responsibilities of nurse and patient are defined.

Goals of the relationship are clarified.

Time and place of meetings are established.

Conditions for termination are outlined.

Confidentiality is discussed and ensured.

---

      c.   Cultural background: distinctive, learned ways of life (e.g., language, customs)

      d.   Roles: social or professional functions (e.g., parent, nurse, student)

4.   Aims of therapeutic communication include:
   a.   Initiating a professional, helpful relationship
   b.   Building trust
   c.   Maintaining a helping relationship over time
   d.   Providing emotional support

5.   Essential elements for therapeutic communication include:
   a.   An unconditionally positive regard for the patient
   b.   Empathy (See Table 1–1 for specific verbal and nonverbal behaviors that convey empathy and nonempathy.)
   c.   Genuineness
   d.   Warmth and respect
   e.   Immediacy
   f.   Purposefulness

6.   Therapeutic communication approaches include:
   a.   Offering self: being available to listen to the patient
   b.   Asking open-ended questions: neutral questions that encourage the patient to express concerns
   c.   Providing opening remarks: general statements based on assessment of the patient
   d.   Restating: repeating to the patient the main content of the communication

TABLE 1–1.
Empathic and Nonempathic Nursing Behaviors

EMPATHIC BEHAVIORS	NONEMPATHIC BEHAVIORS
Focusing on the patient's feelings	Ignoring the patient's feelings
Asking open-ended questions	Asking closed-ended questions
Using a warm vocal tone	Using a flat vocal tone
Conveying a nonjudgmental attitude	Conveying a judgmental attitude
Maintaining eye contact	Looking away
Nodding the head periodically	Nodding too much
Smiling periodically	Picking at clothing
Making smooth gestures	Maintaining facial inexpressiveness
Opening arms	Laughing too much
Leaning forward slightly	Making jerky, stabbing gestures
Appearing comfortable	Crossing arms
Synchronizing movements with those of the patient	Leaning away
	Looking uncomfortable
	Not synchronizing movements with those of the patient

       e.   Reflecting: identifying the main themes contained in a communication and directing these back to the patient

       f.   Focusing: asking goal-directed questions to help the patient focus on a specific content area

       g.   Encouraging elaboration: helping the patient to describe more fully the concerns or problems under discussion

       h.   Seeking clarification: helping the patient put into words unclear thoughts or ideas

       i.   Giving information: sharing with the patient relevant information for his health care and well-being

       j.   Examining alternatives: helping the patient explore options in light of his or her needs and the resources available

       k.   Using silence: allowing periodic pauses in communication to give the nurse and patient time to think about what has taken place

       l.   Summarizing: highlighting the important points of a communication by condensing what has been said or observed

III. Legal and ethical issues

A. Levels of hospital admission

   1.   In *informal admission:*

       a.   Admission is initiated by the patient.

       b.   The patient retains all his civil rights.

       c.   The patient is free to leave at any time.

   2.   In *voluntary admission:*

       a.   Admission is initiated by the patient, a family member, or another on the patient's behalf.

       b.   The patient signs a formal agreement for hospitalization.

       c.   The patient retains all his civil rights.

       d.   A written request must be submitted in order for the patient to leave before discharge.

   3.   In *involuntary admission* (or commitment):

       a.   Admission is ordered by the court, an administrative panel, or a number of physicians.

       b.   The patient has been judged dangerous to himself or herself, dangerous to others, or in need of treatment.

       c.   The patient may or may not retain his or her civil rights (depending on specific state legislation).

       d.   The patient can be hospitalized against his or her will and must be formally discharged in order to leave.

B. Patient rights

   1.   Most psychiatric inpatient units have adopted a Patient Bill of Rights based on one issued by the American Hospital Association in 1973.

   2.   These patient rights include the following:

       a.   The right to communicate with people outside the hospital

      b.   The right to keep clothing and personal effects
      c.   The right to religious freedom, employment, education
      d.   The right to make purchases, manage property
      e.   The right to habeas corpus
      f.   The right to independent psychiatric evaluation and to periodic review of status
      g.   The right to civil service status
      h.   The right to retain licenses (e.g., driver's, professional)
      i.   The right to sue or be sued and to legal representation
      j.   The right not to be subjected to unnecessary mechanical restraints
      k.   The right to privacy
      l.   The right to informed consent and treatment in the least restrictive setting

C.   **Ethical dilemmas commonly faced by nurses**
    1.   What distinguishes eccentric or bizarre behavior from mental illness?
    2.   When can a patient refuse hospitalization, therapy, or medications?
    3.   When should a patient's movement or privileges be restricted?
    4.   When should confidential information be shared?
    5.   When should the nurse intervene to prevent the patient from harming himself or others?

D.   **Legal and ethical responsibilities of nurses**
    1.   Comply with the law.
    2.   Uphold patient rights.
    3.   Clarify personal and professional values.
    4.   Act as an advocate for the mental health needs and rights of patients, families, and the community.

Bibliography

American Nurses' Association (1982). *ANA standards of psychiatric and mental health nursing practice*. Kansas City, MO: American Nurses Association.

Johnson, B. S. (1989). *Psychiatric-mental health nursing: Adaptation and growth* (2nd ed.). Philadelphia: J. B. Lippincott.

Stuart, G., & Sundeen, S. (1987). *Principles and practice of psychiatric nursing* (3rd ed.). St. Louis: C. V. Mosby.

Wilson, H., & Kneisl, C. (1988). *Psychiatric nursing* (3rd ed.). Menlo Park, CA: Addison-Wesley.

STUDY QUESTIONS

1. Below are four descriptions of roles assumed by nurses. Which one represents a role unique to the mental health and psychiatric nurse?
   a. provides direct patient care, including medications, treatments, and promotion of self-care
   b. assists patient to communicate and relate to others more effectively
   c. coordinates diverse aspects of care by working with other health team members
   d. serves as an advocate on behalf of patients and their families

2. All but one of the following statements about a therapeutic nurse–patient relationship are true. Which one is *not* true?
   a. The social needs of both participants are considered.
   b. The relationship is focused on the patient's needs and problems.
   c. The relationship is directed toward specific goals.
   d. The relationship has clearly defined parameters.

3. Getting acquainted and developing trust and open communication characterize which phase of the nurse–patient relationship?
   a. orientation
   b. working
   c. termination
   d. evaluation

4. The overall purpose of therapeutic communication is to
   a. analyze the patient's problems
   b. facilitate and maintain a relationship that is helpful to the patient
   c. provide emotional support during difficult times
   d. ensure that the patient will remain cooperative

5. Whether or not to administer medications to a psychotic patient who refuses them because he or she believes they're poison is an example of which ethical issue?

   a. maintaining role parameters of the nurse–patient relationship
   b. using authority in the nurse–patient relationship
   c. using unconditional positive regard
   d. encountering a conflict of interest over patient rights

6. In the communication process, feedback refers to
   a. response of the receiver to the sender
   b. originator of a message
   c. setting in which communication takes place
   d. information transmitted

7. Which of the following would be an *inappropriate* topic to raise during the orientation phase of the nurse–patient relationship?
   a. the patient's perception of the reason for hospitalization
   b. clarification of the roles of nurse and patient
   c. conditions for termination of the relationship
   d. exploration of the patient's inadequate coping mechanisms

8. A newly admitted patient says, "I just don't know if I should be here. What will my family think?" Using the response of reflection, which of the following statements by the nurse would be most appropriate?
   a. "It's hard to be here; you're concerned about your family's reaction."
   b. "What your family thinks isn't important. It's you that we're concerned about."
   c. "It sounds like your family doesn't understand you."
   d. "You can't always please your family, can you?"

9. Mary Gladstone, RN, is caring for a domineering patient who reminds her of her own rather harsh and demanding mother. At the end of the interaction,

Mary seeks out a colleague with whom she explores her feelings about the patient. This action by Mary indicates
a. inability to cope effectively
b. the presence of dependency needs
c. appropriate self-awareness
d. the need for psychotherapy

10. After having one conversation with a female nurse, a young male patient asks the nurse for her phone number, stating that he would like to date her. Which of the following responses would be most appropriate?
a. "I'm sorry, but I'm married and not interested in dating."
b. "It's against hospital policy for me to date patients."
c. "This is a professional relationship, and we need to stay clear on that."
d. "I may consider dating you once you have fully recovered."

11. The nurse and patient are in the working phase of their relationship. During the interaction, the patient has been talking about some important problems and revealing a lot about himself. Now he falls silent. The best initial nursing action would be to
a. encourage the patient to keep on talking
b. remain silent with the patient, staying attentive
c. ask the patient a nonthreatening question
d. terminate the interaction

12. Mr. Harris was admitted for acute psychosis, manifested by auditory hallucinations and withdrawal. He refuses to take antipsychotic medications because they "make my head feel fuzzy." The staff observes that he is becoming more psychotic without the medications. The health team meets to discuss the problem of Mr. Harris's noncompliance. Which of the following statements made during the discussion reflects consideration for the ethics involved in solving this problem?
a. "Mr. Harris needs the medications

because he's becoming more psychotic. We can give an injectable form and restrain him while giving it. It's for his own good."
b. "Since Mr. Harris needs the medication, we can put a liquid form of it into his orange juice without telling him. He probably won't notice."
c. "Mr. Harris has the right to be psychotic. Let's consider transferring him to a unit where he can be as psychotic as he wants to be."
d. "We need to explore the potential consequences of various options. Let's examine each alternative in light of his situation."

13. Which of the following suggestions made by staff reflects the best potential solution to the problem of Mr. Harris's noncompliance?
a. Have Mr. Harris's family meet with the staff to decide whether or not he should be forced to take his medications.
b. Have Mr. Harris's psychiatrist and primary nurse explore options with him about taking his medications.
c. Discharge Mr. Harris because he does not qualify for commitment proceedings.
d. Take away Mr. Harris's privileges until he complies with his treatment program.

14. A patient hospitalized under a voluntary admission wants to call his lawyer about a personal matter involving a lawsuit with his neighbor. Which of the following nursing actions would be appropriate in this case?
a. Allow the phone call without seeking further information.
b. Ask the patient detailed questions about the lawsuit.
c. Allow the phone call only after the patient explains what the matter is about.
d. Call the lawyer to tell him that his patient is hospitalized.

15. The ANA Standards of Practice for the

nurse who is not Master's or Doctorally prepared include
a. basing actions on theoretic foundations
b. being accountable to a psychiatrist for patient care
c. conducting clinical research
d. conducting psychotherapy

ANSWER KEY

1. *Correct response: b*
   Psychiatric nursing is an interpersonal process aimed at promoting effective communication and interpersonal relationships. Primary work in the interpersonal area is unique to psychiatric nursing.
   a, c, and d. These responsibilities apply to all areas of nursing.
   Knowledge/Safe Care/Implementation

2. *Correct response: a*
   The therapeutic relationship differs from a social one because it is based on the needs of the patient, is goal-directed, and has clear parameters. It is a professional relationship, with the nurse functioning as a therapeutic agent.
   b, c, and d. All of these statements regarding a therapeutic relationship are true.
   Knowledge/Safe Care/Planning

3. *Correct response: a*
   During the orientation phase, the introductory and assessment phase of the nurse–patient relationship, a primary task is to establish trust and open communication so that the nurse and patient can begin to work together.
   b and c. Working and termination both are later phases in the nurse–patient relationship.
   d. Evaluation is a task in the termination phase.
   Knowledge/Psychosocial/Assessment

4. *Correct response: b*
   The aim of therapeutic communication is to foster a helping relationship so that the patient can develop more effective communication and coping behavior.
   a, c, and d. None of these tasks reflects the overall aim of therapeutic communication.
   Knowledge/Safe Care/Planning

5. *Correct response: d*
   Power over patients represents the basis

for conflicts of interest over patient rights. The problem of administering medications to a psychotic patient who staff believes needs them is a common ethical problem in psychiatric care.
   a, b, and c. None of these responses specifies the ethics involved in this scenario.
   Comprehensive/Safe Care/Implementation

6. *Correct response: a*
   This question is based on knowledge about the structural model of communication. Communication has five components: sender, message, receiver, feedback, and context. Feedback refers to the response (verbal or nonverbal) of the receiver in a message back to the sender.
   b, c, and d. These are definitions of sender, context, and message, respectively.
   Knowledge/Safe Care/Implementation

7. *Correct response: d*
   The main focus of the orientation phase is on developing trust, open communication, and a working contract. Exploring coping mechanisms can be carried out only after a trusting relationship is established; thus, it is an inappropriate intervention for the orientation phase.
   a, b, and c. These are all appropriate interventions during the orientation phase.
   Knowledge/Psychosocial/Assessment

8. *Correct response: a*
   This is a reflective response in which the nurse indicates to the patient that he or she is aware of what the patient is experiencing. Reflection indicates understanding, empathy, and respect for the patient's feelings.
   b. This statement devalues what the patient feels by negating what he or she has just said.
   c. This statement diverts the conversation from the patient's perspective and feelings.

d. This statement is inappropriate because it provides false reassurance.
Application/Psychosocial/Implementation

9. *Correct response: c*
Self-awareness is a crucial ingredient in therapeutic intervention. Analyzing and sharing perceptions about self in relation to a patient help the nurse work through countertransference feelings, which could adversely affect the therapeutic process.
a and b. Seeking peer consultation when countertransference occurs does not indicate inability to cope or underlying dependence.
d. Seeking out peer assistance indicates the ability to work through one's own issues. However, if the nurse often experiences very strong feelings in relation to patients, this may indicate a need for psychotherapy.
Application/Safe Care/Implementation

10. *Correct response: c*
At the beginning of a professional relationship, it may be necessary to clarify the parameters of the therapeutic relationship.
a and b. These responses avoid the issue of dealing with the nurse–patient relationship.
d. This is an unprofessional response. Because it is likely that the patient is testing the nurse, this response may be very frightening to him. Promising to date a patient also could create problems for the nurse in the future.
Application/Safe Care/Implementation

11. *Correct response: b*
Silence allows the patient to think and gain insight into what has been talked about. The nurse should allow the silence and convey interest and support.
a, c, and d. These actions would be nontherapeutic in the working phase of a relationship.
Application/Psychosocial/Implementation

12. *Correct response: d*
The patient's right to refuse treatment is a complex issue. Staff must weigh the rights of the patient with professional judgment; careful review of all the options will help the staff make a thoughtful decision.
a and b. These represent violations of the patient's rights.
c. This represents a way of avoiding the ethical dilemma by moving the patient elsewhere.
Application/Safe Care/Implementation

13. *Correct response: b*
One way to deal with medication refusal is to help explore such options as lowering the dosage, changing the medication, or attempting to treat the psychosis without medication. Taking the patient's viewpoint seriously by not forcing the medications on him shows respect for the patient and his rights.
a. This could violate the patient's rights to confidentiality.
c. This action avoids dealing with the medication issue.
d. This action would be punitive.
Application/Safe Care/Implementation

14. *Correct response: a*
One of the patient's rights is to manage his or her personal affairs—to make phone calls, send letters, and so forth.
b and c. These responses indicate that the nurse is being too intrusive into the patient's personal affairs.
d. This represents a clear violation of the patient's right to privacy.
Application/Safe Care/Implementation

15. *Correct response: a*
The standards clearly state that practice is to be guided by the use of theory.
b. This response is incorrect, because the ANA standards are focused on independent nursing functions.
c and d. These responses are incorrect because conducting research and doing psychotherapy require a minimum of a Master's degree preparation.
Knowledge/Safe Care/Assessment

Conceptual Frameworks

for Psychiatric Care

I. **Overview**
  A. Description
  B. Purpose
  C. Predominant conceptual models in psychiatric care
II. **Psychodynamic framework**
  A. Focus: intrapsychic processes
  B. Basic concepts: psychosexual development (Freud's theory)
  C. Basic concepts: developmental stages of man (Erikson's theory)
  D. Basic concepts: personality dynamics
  E. Psychodynamic view of mental illness
  F. Psychodynamic treatment
  G. Nursing application
III. **Behavioral framework**
  A. Focus: learned behavior
  B. Basic concepts
  C. Behavioral view of mental illness
  D. Behavior modification therapy
  E. Nursing application
IV. **Interpersonal framework (Sullivan's theory)**
  A. Focus: interpersonal relationships
  B. Basic concepts

C. Interpersonal view of mental illness
  D. Interpersonal treatment
  E. Nursing application
V. **Cognitive framework**
  A. Focus: cognitive processes
  B. Basic concepts
  C. Cognitive view of mental illness
  D. Cognitive treatments
  E. Nursing application
VI. **Humanistic (existential) framework**
  A. Focus: conscious human experiences of the here and now (e.g., Perls', Glasser's, and Rogers' theories)
  B. Basic concepts
  C. Humanistic view of mental illness
  D. Humanistic treatment
  E. Nursing application
VII. **Biomedical framework**
  A. Focus: disease approach
  B. Basic concepts
  C. Biomedical view of mental illness
  D. Biomedical treatment
  E. Nursing application
Bibliography
Study Questions

I. **Overview**
   A. **Description: Conceptual models are frameworks for organizing and better understanding a body of knowledge.**
   B. **Purpose**
      1. Conceptual models help the nurse take a rational, systematic approach to patient care and decision making by:
         a. Providing reasons or explanations for situations and behaviors confronted
         b. Providing rationales for actions to be taken
      2. These models also facilitate research.
   C. **Predominant conceptual models in psychiatric care**
      1. Psychodynamic framework
      2. Behavioral framework
      3. Interpersonal framework
      4. Cognitive framework
      5. Humanistic (or existential) framework
      6. Biomedical framework

II. **Psychodynamic framework**
   A. **Focus: intrapsychic processes**
      1. Conflicts
      2. Anxiety
      3. Defenses
      4. Impulses (e.g., sexual, aggressive)
   B. **Basic concepts: psychosexual development (Freud's theory)**
      1. Oral stage (infancy)
         a. Gratification of basic oral needs
         b. Development of basic trust
      2. Anal stage (toddlerhood)
         a. Exercise of muscle control (e.g., toilet training)
         b. Development of social controls
         c. Development of autonomy
      3. Phallic stage (preschool age)
         a. Sexual interest; gender identification
         b. Oedipus and Electra complexes (attraction to opposite-sex parent; identification with same-sex parent)
      4. Latency stage (school age)
         a. Dormant sexual interest
         b. Focus on mastery of social and cognitive skills
      5. Genital stage (adolescence and young adulthood)
         a. Renewed sexual interest
         b. Relationships with opposite sex
         c. Capacity to love and work
   C. **Basic concepts: developmental stages of man (Erikson's theory)**
      1. Trust vs. mistrust (infancy)
         a. Basic needs fulfillment

      b.   Issues of trust development with significant other
2.   Autonomy vs. shame and doubt (toddlerhood)
      a.   Initial exploration of separation from significant other; independence
      b.   Muscle control (toilet training); other aspects of self-control
3.   Initiative vs. guilt (preschool age)
      a.   Examination of love and hate
      b.   Exploration of action, sense of purpose
4.   Industry vs. inferiority (school age)
      a.   Realization of issues of competence and competition or comparison
      b.   Purposeful work; perseverance tested
5.   Identity vs. identity diffusion (adolescence)
      a.   Exploration of sense of self
      b.   Initial identification of future goals or potentials
6.   Intimacy vs. stagnation (young adulthood)
      a.   Capacity for love and intimacy
      b.   Commitment in relationships and work
7.   Generativity vs. stagnation (middle adulthood)
      a.   Exploration of concern for others over concern for self
      b.   Productivity; leaving a mark on society
8.   Ego integrity vs. despair (later adulthood)
      a.   Adjustment to life transitions
      b.   Life review (evaluation of life)
      c.   Preparation for death

D. **Basic concepts: personality dynamics**
   1.   Components of personality
      a.   Id—pleasure principle: instincts and primitive impulses
      b.   Ego—reality principle: "I" component, must be in touch with reality
      c.   Superego—moral principle: conscience and culturally acquired values
   2.   Levels of consciousness
      a.   Conscious: perceptual awareness
      b.   Preconscious: memories and experiences easily brought into awareness
      c.   Unconscious: memories and experiences barred from awareness
   3.   Defense mechanisms: coping strategies to alleviate anxiety (see Chapter 3 and Table 2–1)

E. **Psychodynamic view of mental illness**
   1.   This framework applies mainly to nonpsychotic conditions.
   2.   Abnormal behavior is traced back to unresolved problems occurring in earlier developmental stages.

TABLE 2-1.
Defense Mechanisms

DEFENSE MECHANISM	CLINICAL EXAMPLE
Repression	An accident victim remembers nothing about his accident.
Projection	A frightened patient lashes out at the nurse, saying the nurse "doesn't know what is going on."
Reaction formation	A patient is angry about the care received but behaves in an ingratiating manner.
Displacement	A patient who is angry at his doctor becomes verbally abusive to the nurses.
Identification	A teenager hospitalized for diabetes wants to become a nurse as a result of his experiences.
Denial	A patient who drinks alcohol every day and cannot stop fails to acknowledge that he has a problem.
Isolation	A rape victim talks about her rape experience without showing any emotion.
Intellectualization	A parent talks with his child about what love should be like but fails to demonstrate love toward the child.
Rationalization	A patient being treated for a drug addiction says he cannot stop taking drugs because he has a "bad marriage."
Sublimation	A mother who lost a son in a drunk-driving accident joins an organization that works to educate the public about the dangers of drunk driving.

3. Anxiety results from repressed developmental conflicts.
4. Psychic energy is invested in defenses that control anxiety related to repressed conflicts.
5. A person behaves in less mature ways because defenses are fixed at an earlier developmental stage.
6. Such a person has difficulty coping effectively with life's circumstances.

F. **Psychodynamic treatment**
   1. Focuses on conflicts, anxiety, defenses, and sexual and aggressive drives
   2. Seeks to alter thought and behavior by examining and resolving earlier conflicts
   3. Makes conscious that which is repressed, through:
      a. Free association
      b. Dream analysis
      c. Transference analysis (analysis of person's feelings about therapist)
      d. Catharsis (uncovering and reliving traumatic events)

G. **Nursing application**
   1. A nurse typically does not conduct psychodynamic therapy unless trained at the postgraduate level.
   2. Principles of psychodynamics often prove useful in interpreting a patient's behavior.

3. Attention is given to a patient's anxiety and defensive behaviors.
4. A nurse commonly performs developmental assessment using Erikson's developmental stages.

III. Behavioral framework

A. Focus: learned behavior

1. Persons are shaped by their environment.
2. Various behaviors are subject to reward or punishment.
3. Experiments can determine what environmental aspects affect behavior.
4. Certain behaviors can be changed if the environment is changed.

B. Basic concepts

1. Classical conditioning (Pavlov's theory) Dogs
    a. Conditioning response: pairing of stimulus with response
    b. Acquisition: gain of a learned behavioral response
    c. Extinction: loss of a learned response
2. Operant conditioning (Skinner's theory) Rat
    a. Positive reinforcer: reward for a behavior that will help continue the behavior
    b. Negative reinforcer: punishment for a behavior that will discourage the behavior
    c. Operant behavior: behavior that can be reinforced

C. Behavioral view of mental illness

1. This framework applies mainly to anxiety disorders, phobias, and behavioral problems.
2. Maladaptive behaviors are learned through classical and operant problems.
3. Maladaptive behaviors are maintained through reinforcement.
4. Maladaptive behaviors can be modified by changing the environment.
5. The environment can be changed by altering original stimuli and using positive or negative reinforcers.

D. Behavior modification therapy

1. The basic process involves:
    a. Targeting maladaptive behavior by specifically defining it
    b. Identifying reinforcers that help maintain maladaptive behavior
    c. Identifying adaptive behavior to replace maladaptive behavior
    d. Identifying reinforcers that will discourage undesirable behavior and encourage desirable behavior
    e. Substituting one stimulus with another

2. Types of treatment include:
   a. Systematic desensitization: gradually confronting a situation that evokes anxiety
   b. Flooding: immersing oneself in a situation that evokes anxiety
   c. Aversive therapy: applying an unpleasant stimulus (e.g., electric shock) to discourage a maladaptive behavior
   d. Biofeedback: training to control physiologic responses
   e. Relaxation techniques: training to counteract nervous tension
   f. Assertiveness training: training to overcome passivity in interpersonal situations

E. **Nursing application**
   1. The nurse applies behavioral principles in inpatient psychiatric care.
   2. Techniques for limit setting are based on behavioral principles.
   3. The nurse and patient collaborate in identifying target behaviors for modification.
   4. Privileges such as phone use and off-unit movement are used as reinforcers.
   5. The patient practices new behaviors with the nurse's help.
   6. Homework and reinforcement exercises are often used.

IV. **Interpersonal framework (Sullivan's theory)**
   A. **Focus: interpersonal relationships**
      1. Personality development results from interaction with significant other(s).
      2. The child internalizes approval or disapproval by significant others, creating his or her self-concept (or "self-system").

   B. **Basic concepts**
      1. Human beings have two basic drives:
         a. Satisfaction: basic needs for food, rest, sex, relatedness
         b. Security: culturally defined needs for conformity, similarity of values
      2. A person's degree of satisfaction and security reflects positive or negative relationships.
      3. Anxiety plays a crucial role in personality development and later coping; anxiety is related to disapproval.
      4. A crucial link exists between thought and language; verbal sharing in a relationship clarifies thinking and reduces anxiety.

   C. **Interpersonal view of mental illness**
      1. Three personifications of "me" can evolve through relationships with significant others:
         a. "Good me," resulting from positive approval and leading to good feelings about self
         b. "Bad me," resulting from experiences related to increased anxiety and leading to anxiety states

      c.   "Not me," resulting from very disapproving messages and leading to overwhelming anxiety

    2.   Security operations become a part of responding or coping to help the person avoid or minimize anxiety.

    3.   If anxiety is great, the person is unable to evaluate self objectively.

    4.   If anxiety is great, the person also cannot operate in a mature (syntactic) mode of experiencing.

  D. **Interpersonal treatment**

    1.   A trusting, therapeutic relationship is the basis for a corrective experience.

    2.   The patient is encouraged to share anxieties and feelings with the therapist.

    3.   The therapist assists the patient in developing close relationships.

  E. **Nursing application**

    1.   Hildegaard Peplau, a renowned nurse theorist, developed an interpersonal theory of nursing using Sullivan's ideas.

    2.   Nursing focuses on the nurse–patient relationship, the vehicle through which the patient becomes healthy.

    3.   Nurses counsel patients by developing a therapeutic relationship.

    4.   Counseling performed by nurses tends to focus on "here-and-now" interpersonal concerns.

    5.   Anxiety intervention is an important nursing role (see Chapter 3).

    6.   Nurses assist psychiatric patients with effective problem solving related to interpersonal issues.

    7.   Nurses use the nurse–patient relationship as a corrective interpersonal experience for patients.

V. **Cognitive framework**

  A. **Focus: cognitive processes**

    1.   Cognitive processes include expectations, beliefs, memory, and thinking patterns.

    2.   Thinking influences feelings and behavior.

  B. **Basic concepts**

    1.   Cognitive processes can be altered or restructured.

    2.   Appraisals are the automatic thoughts a person uses to evaluate his or her present situation.

    3.   Attributions refer to a person's conception of why an event is happening. They may be:

        a.   External, arising from outside the self

        b.   Internal, arising from within the self

    4.   Beliefs are long-held ideas that shape thoughts, feelings, and behavior.

    C.   **Cognitive view of mental illness**
        1.   This framework is especially applicable to depression but also is useful in addressing other mental disorders.
        2.   Distorted thinking (e.g., irrational and illogical beliefs, unrealistic self-appraisals, and rigid attributions) causes disordered behavior.

    D.   **Cognitive treatment**
        1.   The basic process involves:
            a.   Identifying cognitive processes by listening to the patient
            b.   Making the patient aware of cognitive processes
            c.   Disputing cognitive processes that underlie maladaptive feelings and behaviors
            d.   Encouraging the patient to practice alternative thought patterns
        2.   Types of treatment include:
            a.   Rational-emotive therapy (Ellis): disputes underlying irrational beliefs
            b.   Multimodal therapy (Lazarus): separates the disorder into different levels and applies various techniques
            c.   Cognitive therapy: teaches the patient new cognitive structures (cognitive restructuring)

    E.   **Nursing application**
        1.   Nurses assess patients' thought (cognitive) patterns.
        2.   Nurses participate in cognitive restructuring as part of a team approach.
        3.   At the graduate level, nurses may learn cognitive therapy.

VI.   **Humanistic (existential) framework**
    A.   **Focus: conscious human experiences of the here and now (e.g., Perls', Glasser's, and Rogers' theories)**
        1.   Human beings have the potential to grow.
        2.   Human beings can exercise freedom of choice.
        3.   Freedom to choose among alternatives gives meaning to a person's life.
        4.   Human beings are responsible for their own behavior.

    B.   **Basic concepts**
        1.   Human existence is a search for meaning, authenticity, and realization of potential.
        2.   Human needs are organized in a hierarchy (Maslow's theory), ranging from biologic needs to self-actualization.
        3.   As a person's basic needs are gratified, higher-level needs emerge.
        4.   If lower-level needs are not satisfied, insecurity and regression occur.
        5.   When basic needs are met, a person becomes growth-oriented.

C. **Humanistic view of mental illness**
1. Mental illness is an alienation from self that hinders freedom of choice, responsibility, and growth.
2. Lack of self-awareness and unmet needs interfere with relationships and with feelings of security.
3. The fundamental human anxiety is the fear of death.
4. Recovery involves heightened awareness of being and of potential for growth, love, and fulfillment.

D. **Humanistic treatment**
1. In *client-centered therapy* (Rogers):
   a. The patient experiences the therapist's unconditional positive regard and respect.
   b. The therapist attempts to achieve empathic rapport with the patient.
   c. The therapist listens carefully to the patient and reflects what is understood.
   d. The patient develops self-understanding through the process of being accepted and understood.
   e. This self-understanding leads to awareness of choice and responsibility.
2. In *gestalt therapy* (Perls):
   a. The patient is assisted to express feelings directly.
   b. Various techniques, such as role playing, are used to act out past experiences and feelings.
   c. Confronting feelings leads to acceptance of self.
   d. Acceptance of self leads to more mature behavior.

E. **Nursing application**
1. Basic nurse–patient interactions are based on humanistic principles, such as:
   a. Positive regard
   b. Empathy
   c. Respect
2. Nurse–patient interactions are client-centered, in which:
   a. The patient is encouraged to initiate topics of concern.
   b. The nurse listens carefully to the patient.
   c. The nurse uses reflective listening approaches to help the patient gain self-understanding.
   d. The nurse helps the patient examine alternative choices.

VII. **Biomedical framework**
A. **Focus: disease approach**
1. Identification of syndromes (diverse symptoms occurring together)
2. Establishment of diagnoses
3. Search for etiologies (e.g., bacterial or viral infection, genetic transmission, biochemistry)

B. **Basic concepts**
   1. Physiologic, social, or environmental factors cause or predispose to mental illness.
   2. Mental illnesses have certain symptoms that can be classified and treated.
   3. The mentally ill patient assumes the sick role.
   4. Evidence supporting the biomedical approach to mental illness includes:
      a. Eradication of general paresis (tertiary syphilis) through the discovery of causative bacteria
      b. Presence of genetic transmission patterns in schizophrenia and affective disorders
      c. Reduction of symptoms through the use of pharmaceutical agents

C. **Biomedical view of mental illness**
   1. Mental illness is a disorder of the body.
   2. Mental illnesses can be classified, as in the *Diagnostic and Statistical Manual of Mental Disorders,* 3rd edition revised (DSM-III-R).
   3. Labeling a mental disorder as an illness helps the patient and family focus on treatment and recovery.

D. **Biomedical treatment**
   1. Diagnostic workups include detailed history and laboratory tests as well as careful observation of current behavior.
   2. Pharmacotherapy is a common treatment.
   3. The physician–patient relationship is fostered to engender trust and compliance with the treatment regimen.
   4. Psychotherapy has become part of the biomedical model.

E. **Nursing application**
   1. Nurses work in biomedically oriented settings.
   2. Nursing is one of the four core psychiatric disciplines identified by the National Institutes of Mental Health (*i.e.,* physician, nurse, psychologist, social worker).
   3. Nurses observe and assess patient behavior as well as facilitate physical well-being.
   4. Nurses administer treatments and foster patient compliance.
   5. Nurses teach patients about their illnesses, including:
      a. Recognition of symptoms
      b. Management of illness
      c. Prevention of relapse
   6. Nurses coordinate diverse aspects of care.
   7. Nurses act as patient advocates within the biomedical health care system.
   8. Nurses prepared at the graduate level or above can participate in assessing patients for DSM-III-R diagnosis and also can conduct psychotherapy.

Bibliography

Johnson, B. S. (1989). *Psychiatric-mental health nursing: Adaptation and growth* (2nd ed.). Philadelphia: J. B. Lippincott.

Rosenham, D. L., & Seligman, M. E. (1984). *Abnormal psychology.* New York: W. W. Norton.

Smith, R. E., Sarason, I. G., & Sarason, B. R. (1982). *Psychology: The frontiers of behavior.* New York: Harper & Row.

Stuart, G., & Sundeen, S. (1987). *Principles and practice of psychiatric nursing* (3rd ed.). St. Louis: C. V. Mosby.

Wilson, H., & Kneisl, C. (1988). *Psychiatric nursing* (3rd ed.). Menlo Park, CA: Addison-Wesley.

STUDY QUESTIONS

1. As a consistent aspect of the care environment, the staff meets weekly to discuss the diagnoses and treatment protocols of newly admitted patients. Which framework for psychiatric care does this approach represent?
   a. biomedical
   b. psychodynamic
   c. behavioral
   d. cognitive

2. The patient's problems and behaviors are interpreted in terms of anxiety and repressed conflicts. Which framework for psychiatric care does this approach represent?
   a. biomedical
   b. psychodynamic
   c. behavioral
   d. cognitive

3. A patient newly diagnosed with cancer fails to talk about or acknowledge the diagnosis, acting as if nothing is wrong. Which defense mechanism is this patient using?
   a. projection
   b. identification
   c. rationalization
   d. denial

4. In planning a patient's care, the nursing staff identifies privileges (e.g., use of telephone, participation in recreational activities) to be used as rewards for desirable behavior. These privileges serve as a (an)
   a. extinction
   b. response
   c. operant
   d. reinforcer

5. The *Diagnostic and Statistical Manual of Mental Disorders,* 3rd edition revised (DSM-III-R) mainly provides
   a. treatment protocols for mental disorders
   b. epidemiologic information about mental disorders
   c. classification and diagnostic criteria for mental disorders

   d. rates of severity of mental disorders according to statistical information

6. Listening carefully as the patient talks about his choices and responsibilities in life reflects which framework for psychiatric care?
   a. biomedical
   b. humanistic
   c. behavioral
   d. cognitive

7. During assessment, a patient says to the nurse, "I don't know what to do. My marriage is terrible, and I just got fired from my job." Of the responses below, which one is client-centered?
   a. "Your thoughts are negative right now and this keeps you from making decisions."
   b. "Things in your life are not working well right now and you feel unsure about what to do."
   c. "Have you considered marriage counseling? Many people find that helpful."
   d. "Other people have difficulties too. Have you shared these feelings with others?"

8. The primary nurse encourages a patient to record her ongoing thoughts in a daily diary. The nurse then reviews the diary with the patient in order to identify thought patterns that appear to contribute to the patient's feelings of depression and anxiety. This nursing intervention is based on which framework for psychiatric care?
   a. biomedical
   b. psychodynamic
   c. behavioral
   d. cognitive

9. Based on Maslow's theory, which human need must be met first before the others can be considered?
   a. security and safety
   b. love and acceptance
   c. beauty and philosophy
   d. recognition and competence

10. Barney, a retarded and emotionally disturbed young man, is admitted to a unit for patients with unsocialized, aggressive behavior. Even though he has the capabilities, he refuses to bathe, eat with utensils, or participate in structured activities. He carries a teddy bear with him at all times and screams relentlessly if a staff member tries to take the bear away from him. He looks forward to his parents' weekly visits, and he has made some friends on the unit. A plan of care based on behavioral principles is designed for Barney. What would a behaviorist be likely to say about Barney's unsocialized, aggressive behavior?
   a. It has been reinforced so that it continues.
   b. It needs to be punished so that it stops.
   c. It is too extreme to be modified.
   d. It is untreatable because he is retarded.

11. Using careful observation, the staff lists Barney's problematic behaviors. The list includes in what situations the behaviors occur, how long they last, and what happens immediately before and after the behaviors. This procedure is used to
   a. enable Barney to gain insight into his behaviors
   b. define behaviors that are targeted for change
   c. develop a method for desensitizing Barney

   d. eventually confront Barney with his behavior

12. Based on the information given, which reinforcer would best modify Barney's behavior?
   a. structured activities
   b. time with friends
   c. the teddy bear
   d. visits from his parents

13. A 5-year-old girl wants to spend extra time with her "daddy." According to Freud's developmental theory, she is exhibiting
   a. latency phase
   b. oedipal conflict
   c. oral needs
   d. anal patterns

14. Which part of the personality houses primitive drives and operates on the pleasure principle?
   a. id
   b. ego
   c. superego
   d. alterego

15. A man released from prison for selling narcotics has been rehabilitated and now works for an agency that educates youths on the dangers of drug use. This man's current behavior reflects which of the following defense mechanisms?
   a. displacement
   b. identification
   c. denial
   d. sublimation

ANSWER KEY

1. Correct response: a

The biomedical framework is based on the disease model. Syndromes are diagnosed and treatment plans are based on what is currently known about the condition and its treatment.

b, c, and d. These responses refer to other frameworks for psychiatric practice.

Comprehension/Safe care/Planning

2. Correct response: b

Psychodynamic interpretations are based on the idea that repressed conflicts and drives, when not worked through at prior developmental levels, create anxiety. When anxiety is great enough, symptoms of mental disorder occur.

a, c, and d. These responses refer to other frameworks for psychiatric care.

Comprehension/Safe care/Assessment

3. Correct response: d

Failure to acknowledge a problem can be a form of denial. This commonly happens in the earlier stages of a serious diagnosis and occurs so that the ego will not be overwhelmed with anxiety.

a, b, and c. These are other defense mechanisms.

Comprehension/Psychosocial/Assessment

4. Correct response: d

A reinforcer increases the likelihood that a behavior will reoccur. In this instance, staff wants to increase desirable behaviors by using privileges to reward them.

a. Extinction refers to withholding reinforcement so that the behaviors decrease.

b. Response refers to a behavior directly resulting from a stimulus.

c. Operant refers to a specific behavior.

Comprehension/Psychosocial/Planning

5. Correct response: c

The DSM-III-R is used by the four core disciplines in psychiatry to diagnose mental disorders both nationally and internationally.

a and d. This information is not provided in DSM-III-R.

b. This is only partially true; some epidemiologic information is provided by the DSM-III-R, but it is scant.

Knowledge/Health Promotion/Assessment

6. Correct response: b

The humanistic framework focuses on individual choice and responsibility. The focus of psychiatric care from this framework is on being client-centered. From the humanistic perspective, the nurse waits for the client to introduce his concerns.

a, c, and d. These responses refer to other frameworks.

Comprehension/Psychosocial/Implementation

7. Correct response: b

Client-centered responses are based on active listening techniques. In this example, the nurse reflects to the patient what she heard him say. Client-centered responses help the patient to understand himself better.

a. This response is incorrect because the nurse focuses on the patient's cognitive processes.

c and d. These responses are incorrect because the nurse ignores the patient's feelings by suggesting that the patient discuss them with someone else.

Application/Psychosocial/Implementation

8. Correct response: d

The cognitive approach is based on the idea that thoughts influence behavior and feelings. In this example, the patient must first identify recurrent thought processes that cause her to stay depressed and anxious. Cognitive approaches are especially effective with depressed patients.

a, b, and c. These responses refer to

other frameworks for psychiatric care.

Application/Psychosocial/Implementation

9. *Correct response: a*

 After food and water, security and safety are necessary before a person can strive to meet higher needs. Physiologic needs take precedence over psychologic and spiritual needs.

 b, c, and d. These all are higher needs on Maslow's hierarchy.

Knowledge/Physiologic/Assessment

10. *Correct response: a*

 Stimuli in the environment are keeping Barney's behavior in place. For example, if no one bothers him when he is aggressive, or no demands are placed on him because he is uncooperative, leaving him alone serves as a reinforcement because Barney does not have to comply.

 b. Punishment is a simplistic and possibly harmful approach to the problem. Punishment should be used only as a last resort in a behavioral approach.

 c and d. Extreme behaviors in retarded persons have been successfully treated with behavioral treatment programs.

Analysis/Psychosocial/Assessment

11. *Correct response: b*

 Before behavioral strategies are implemented, the target behaviors—those needing to be changed—must be clearly identified.

 a. This is not the behaviorist's primary purpose for documenting patient's behaviors. Insight is not a goal of behavioral intervention. In addition, Barney does not have the capacity for insight.

 c. Desensitization is not the treatment of choice in this case.

 d. This approach is not based on behavioral principles.

Analysis/Safe care/Assessment

12. *Correct response: c*

 The fact that Barney screams relentlessly when the teddy bear is taken from him

shows that this is a very important source of gratification for him. Barney becomes aggressive when the teddy bear is removed. He could be told that he must be cooperative for specified amounts of time without the teddy bear. When he complies with this demand, the teddy bear is given to him as a reward. The amounts of time can be gradually lengthened and other rewards can be introduced.

 a. Barney does not want to participate in structured activities.

 b and d. These items are not as important or as immediate to Barney and therefore would not be adequate reinforcers.

Analysis/Psychosocial/Planning

13. *Correct response: b*

 According to Freud's theory of psychosexual development, girls experience sexual feelings toward their fathers (and boys toward their mothers) around ages 3 to 5 years. Oedipal conflict refers to having feelings of attachment for the parent of the opposite sex and feelings of envy and aggression toward the parent of the same sex.

 a, c, and d. These responses refer to other phases in Freud's developmental theory.

Comprehension/Psychosocial/Assessment

14. *Correct response: a*

 In psychoanalytic theory, id refers to that part of the personality that contains primitive drives.

 b. The ego deals with reality.

 c. The superego is associated with values, ethics, and conscience.

 d. Alterego is not considered part of the basic personality structure.

Knowledge/Psychosocial/NA

15. *Correct response: d*

 Sublimation is a defense in which socially unacceptable drives are converted into socially acceptable avenues.

 a, b, and c. These are other defense mechanisms.

Comprehension/Psychosocial/Assessment

Stress, Anxiety, and Anxiety-Related Disorders

I. Overview of stress

A. Definitions

1. Stress: demands made on a person that exceed the person's coping resources and abilities, causing an adverse affect

2. Stressors: sources or causes of stress; demanding life situations

B. Basic concepts
1. Stress is always present.
2. Stress is more evident during periods of transition and rapid change.
3. Stress can motivate and challenge a person.
4. Severe stress can deplete reserve physiologic capacity and predispose to illness.
5. Common coping measures for stress reduction include:
    a. Turning to a supportive person
    b. Displaying self-discipline and perseverance
    c. Exhibiting intense expressions of emotion (e.g., crying, laughing, yelling)
    d. Ventilating
    e. Privately thinking through options
    f. "Working it off" through purposeful or nonpurposeful activity

C. Etiology
1. Stressors may be physiologic, chemical, developmental, emotional, cognitive, or external events.
2. Stressors may arise from life events.
3. Life events that create stress can be positive or negative. Examples include:
    a. Getting married
    b. Taking out a loan
    c. Having a baby
    d. Getting fired from a job
    e. Getting a job promotion
4. Life events that require adaptation can increase a person's vulnerability to physical illness or ability to deal with further stress.
5. The greater the number of stressful life events, the more likely a person is to develop physical illness or a coping deficit.

II. Nursing process and stress
A. Assessment
1. Note subjective symptoms of stress, such as:
    a. Anxiety
    b. Fatigue
    c. Physical illness
    d. Substance abuse
2. Assess for common clinical manifestations of excessive stress, which reflect response to the fight (aggression)-or-flight (withdrawal) reaction and may include:
    a. Increased heart rate
    b. Elevated blood pressure
    c. Rapid, shallow respirations

      d. Heightened senses
      e. Dilated pupils
      f. Increased muscle tension
      g. Increased perspiration

B. **Nursing diagnoses**
1. Ineffective Individual Coping
2. Diversional Activity Deficit
3. Altered Health Maintenance
4. Nutrition, Altered: Less or More than Body Requirements
5. Sleep Pattern Disturbance

C. **Planning and implementation: stress management**
1. Help the patient develop awareness of stressors.
2. Teach the patient to monitor his or her own physical responses to stress.
3. Help the patient monitor general body tension.
4. Help the patient become aware of psychologic responses to stress.
5. Promote relaxation.
6. Teach breathing techniques to aid stress reduction, including:
    a. Awareness of breathing pattern (should be deep and even)
    b. Deep breathing, using the diaphragm and inhaling through the nose and exhaling through the mouth
    c. Ten-to-one count: inhaling with a deep breath, then exhaling slowly, counting down from 10 to 0 and saying with each number, "I feel more relaxed than at the previous number."
    d. Alternate-nostril breathing: closing right nostril with right thumb and inhaling slowly and deeply through left nostril, then releasing right nostril and closing left nostril with right index finger and exhaling through right nostril; repeating for left side, then alternating sides.
7. Teach relaxation techniques, such as:
    a. Active progressive relaxation: tensing each of four muscle groups (hands, forearms, and biceps; head, face, throat, and shoulders; chest, abdomen, and lower back; thighs, buttocks, calves, and feet) for 10 to 15 seconds, then relaxing for 20 to 30 seconds
    b. Passive progressive relaxation: consciously relaxing muscles without first tensing them, starting with the toes and moving systematically up the body to the head
    c. Music therapy: listening to music that has a relaxing effect; varies among individuals
8. Teach visualization for relaxation and for symptom control.
9. Teach about biofeedback, the ability to gain voluntary control over some autonomic functions with the assistance of a monitoring device.

D. Evaluation

1. The patient states awareness of stressors.
2. The patient reports precipitating stressors absent, reduced, or managed.

III. Overview of anxiety

A. Definition: vague feelings of apprehension, terror, or dread arising from identified or unidentified stressors

B. Basic concepts

1. Anxiety is a universal experience.
2. Anxiety occurs in degrees on a continuum (Fig. 3–1); these degrees include:
   a. Mild
   b. Moderate
   c. Severe
   d. Panic
3. Anxiety often is a motivating force and can provide energy to act.

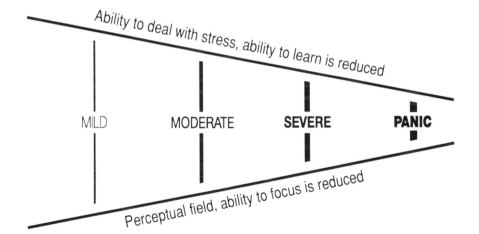

Mild: Increased alertness, enhanced learning ability, enhanced stress management, maximized problem-solving.

Moderate: Ability to focus on central concerns, but more difficulty staying attentive and being able to learn; selective inattention; problem-solving possible with assistance; relaxation techniques helpful.

Severe: Inability to focus or problem-solve, sympathetic nervous system activated; needs structured activities and large muscle activities.

Panic: Complete inability to focus, disintegrated ability to cope; environmental stimuli should be decreased, direction and structure should be provided.

FIGURE 3–1.
Degrees of Anxiety and Their Effects

4. In other cases, anxiety can be so severe as to be immobilizing.
5. Anxiety is not directly observable but rather must be inferred from behavioral and physiologic manifestations.
6. Anxiety is communicable to some degree.
7. Anxiety may be indistinguishable from fear through observation. Fear usually has a specific focus, whereas anxiety typically is more vague. Fear is appropriate to the situation; anxiety may not be rational.

C. Etiology

1. Threats to physical integrity (e.g., impending surgery, physical trauma, lack of essential resources) are common sources of anxiety.
2. Anxiety also may arise from threats to self-concept (e.g., losses, role changes, decreased capacity to manage activities of daily living).
3. Individual vulnerability (e.g., oversensitivity, previous experiences, coping difficulties) can predispose to anxiety.

D. Characteristics of anxiety

1. Physiologic manifestations of anxiety primarily involve autonomic nervous system responses, such as:
    a. Increased heart rate
    b. Increased blood pressure
    c. Difficulty breathing
    d. Sweaty palms
    e. Trembling
    f. Dry mouth
    g. Upset stomach
    h. Tightness in throat
2. Common behavioral manifestations of anxiety include:
    a. Irritability
    b. Anger
    c. Withdrawal
    d. Restlessness
    e. Crying
    f. Complaints of dizziness, nervousness, tension
3. Common coping mechanisms (defense mechanisms) for anxiety reduction include:
    a. Denial: blocking out painful or threatening information or feelings
    b. Displacement: shifting of feelings from a person or object to a more neutral person or object
    c. Identification: taking on ideas and behaviors of an admired person
    d. Introjection: taking into one's own personality another's values, opinions, and behaviors

    e.   Intellectualization: avoiding feelings or emotions with excessive reasoning or logic

    f.   Projection: attributing one's own unacceptable thoughts and feelings to another

    g.   Rationalization: providing a socially acceptable or logical explanation for one's own behavior

    h.   Reaction formation: developing an opinion or behavior that is opposite to the true feelings or motivation

    i.   Repression: unconscious exclusion of painful, unacceptable feelings from awareness or memory

    j.   Sublimation: substituting a socially acceptable activity for an unacceptable or blocked drive or emotion

    k.   Suppression: conscious exclusion of painful, unacceptable feelings from awareness or memory

IV. Anxiety-related disorders

A. Panic disorder

1. Description: unpredictable, recurrent attacks of intense anxiety that interfere with normal functioning; commonly associated with agoraphobia

2. Attacks are not associated with an identifiable stimulus but may become associated with specific situations.

3. Anticipatory anxiety, a common complication, leads to avoidance of anxiety-provoking situations.

4. More common in women, this disorder typically starts in early adulthood.

B. Generalized anxiety disorder

1. Description: pervasive, persistent anxiety of at least 6 months' duration

2. This disorder is marked by chronic, persistent feelings of apprehension and dread with no specific identifiable cause.

C. Obsessive-compulsive disorder

1. Obsession: a recurring, disturbing thought that cannot be dismissed from awareness

2. Compulsion: an uncontrollable, persistent behavior of ritualistic nature (e.g., repetitive hand washing, constant straightening of things)

3. Obsessions and compulsions often occur together and can disrupt normal activities.

D. Phobic disorder

1. Description: persistent, irrational fear of a specific object, activity, or situation

2. Intense anxiety occurs from encountering the feared object, activity, or situation.

3. The person recognizes that the fear is irrational but feels powerless to control it.

    4. Examples include:
- a. Agoraphobia: fear of being alone or in public places
- b. Social phobia: fear of potentially embarrassing social situations
- c. Simple phobia: fear of specific things, such as elevators, heights, cats, insects, or snakes

E. Post-traumatic stress syndrome
1. Description: recurrently experienced thoughts and feelings associated with a severe, specific trauma (e.g., combat experiences, rape, serious accident, severe deprivation, torture)
2. Common symptoms include nightmares, flashbacks, intense anxiety, and anger.
3. The syndrome may be acute or can be delayed and become chronic.

F. Somatization disorder
1. Description: a history of multiple physiologic complaints with no associated demonstrable organic pathology
2. The affected person commonly seeks medical attention

G. Conversion disorder
1. Description: loss of or altered physical function suggesting a physiologic disorder but caused by psychologic factors
2. Examples include paralysis, blindness, anesthesia, and coordination disturbance.
3. Unconscious, not intentional, mental processes are involved.
4. Symptoms may be alleviated through self-awareness of underlying psychologic conflict or need.

H. Hypochondriasis
1. Description: preoccupation with the fear of serious disease
2. No physiologic evidence of any organic problem is evident.
3. Even a physician's reassurance of no symptoms does not alleviate the person's fear.

I. Multiple personality disorder
1. Description: existence of two or more distinct personalities within a person
2. These personalities take full control of the person one at a time.
3. The various personalities may or may not be aware of each other.
4. This disorder nearly always is preceded by severe sexual, emotional, or physical abuse in childhood.

J. Psychogenic fugue
1. Description: sudden, unexpected travel away from home with an inability to recall the past
2. It may involve assumption of new identity (partial or complete).
3. Fugue commonly follows severe psychosocial stress, is of brief duration (hours to days), and usually entails full recovery.

K. **Psychogenic amnesia**
1. Description: sudden inability to recall important personal information
2. Memory impairment may be partial or almost complete.
3. Amnesia typically follows severe psychosocial stress; it can accompany post-traumatic stress syndrome.

L. **Depersonalization disorder**
1. Description: altered self-perception in which one's own reality is temporarily lost or changed
2. It involves feelings of detachment; reality testing remains intact.
3. The experience is distressing for the person.

V. **Nursing process in anxiety-related disorders**
A. Assessment
1. Assess for physiologic responses indicating anxiety, including:
   a. Cardiovascular: palpitations, elevated blood pressure, faintness
   b. Respiratory: rapid shallow respirations, shortness of breath, chest pressure, lump in throat
   c. Neuromuscular: hyperreflexia, twitching eyelid, insomnia, tremors, fidgeting, pacing, clumsiness
   d. Gastrointestinal: anorexia, abdominal discomfort or pain, nausea, heartburn, diarrhea
   e. Urinary tract: pressure to urinate, frequency of urination
   f. Skin: flushed face, sweaty palms, itching, hot or cold spells, generalized sweating
2. Note any characteristic behavioral responses, such as:
   a. Restlessness and physical tension
   b. Rapid speech
   c. Lack of coordination
   d. Accident proneness
   e. Interpersonal withdrawal
   f. Inhibition
   g. Avoidance
   h. Compulsive repetitive behavior
3. Note any cognitive responses to anxiety, which may include:
   a. Impaired attention
   b. Poor concentration
   c. Preoccupation
   d. Thought-blocking
   e. Diminished productivity
   f. Self-consciousness
   g. Fears (e.g., of losing control, of injury, of death, of social scrutiny)
4. Observe for affective responses to anxiety, such as:
   a. Uneasiness

      b.   Tenseness

      c.   Fearfulness

      d.   Irritability, edginess

B. **Analysis and nursing diagnoses**

   1.   When differentiating among anxiety responses, the nurse should be aware that:

      a.   The response can be normal and related to specific stressors.

      b.   The response can be out of proportion to the threat.

      c.   The response can be abnormal and be classified as a disorder.

      d.   The nurse's own anxiety must be separated from that of the patient.

   2.   Accurate analysis depends on in-depth data regarding the patient's anxiety, stressors, and past coping experiences.

   3.   Diagnoses of anxiety can be formulated for patients in any clinical setting; examples include:

      a.   Anxiety

         (1)   Related to conflicts

         (2)   Related to environmental stressors

         (3)   Related to severe, specific trauma

      b.   Ineffective Individual Coping

         (1)   Related to environmental stressors

         (2)   Related to developmental coping deficits

         (3)   Related to poor social skills

      c.   Fear

         (1)   Related to specific phobias

         (2)   Related to performing in public

         (3)   Related to being the focus of attention of others

      d.   Self-Esteem Disturbance

C. **Planning and implementation**

   1.   For the patient with severe or panic level anxiety:

      a.   Establish a supportive, trusting relationship.

      b.   Stay with and attempt to calm the patient.

      c.   Keep demands at a level the patient can handle.

      d.   Do not confront the patient about coping mechanisms.

      e.   Convey calmness and give reassurance.

      f.   Limit environmental stimuli.

      g.   Encourage the patient to engage in physical activity to release energy.

      h.   Administer prescribed tranquilizers in a timely manner.

   2.   For the patient with moderate anxiety:

      a.   Teach about precipitating stressors, coping strategies, adaptive and maladaptive responses.

      b.   Use the problem-solving process to help the patient recognize onset of own anxiety, situational stressors, and coping abilities.

    c.   Promote relaxation responses.

3.   For the patient with obsessive-compulsive disorder:

    a.   Allow time to perform ritualistic behaviors. (The patient's anxiety will increase if time is not allowed for compulsive behaviors.)

    b.   Help to set limits on ritualistic behaviors.

    c.   Channel the need to conduct rituals into more socially useful behaviors (e.g., cleaning up after meals instead of repetitive scrubbing of a wall).

    d.   Do not confront the patient about maladaptive behaviors.

    e.   Promote expression of feelings when anxiety is reduced.

    f.   Assess for skin changes if the patient engages in repetitive hand washing. (Provide lotions and mild soaps; plastic gloves may be used to protect hands.)

4.   For the patient with phobias:

    a.   Do not force contact with the phobic object or situation.

    b.   Help the patient to describe what precipitates response to the phobic object.

    c.   Talk with the patient about the phobic object or situation.

    d.   Assist the patient to develop a plan (such as a desensitization program) for confronting the phobic object or situation.

5.   For the patient with somatic complaints or somatoform disorder:

    a.   Convey your understanding that the symptoms are real to the patient, even though no organic pathology is found.

    b.   Provide for dependency needs by being available to the patient.

    c.   Encourage independent behaviors.

    d.   Encourage the patient to verbalize fears and anxieties.

    e.   Discourage verbalization about physical symptoms by minimizing them and not responding with positive reinforcement.

    f.   Report and assess any new physical complaint, because organic pathology is also a possibility in these patients.

    g.   Teach relaxation exercises.

    h.   Administer antianxiety medications as prescribed.

    i.   Divert the patient into constructive activities.

6.   For the patient with dissociative disorder:

    a.   Develop a trusting relationship and provide support during times of depersonalization, emergence of a new personality, or amnesia.

    b.   Encourage disclosure of painful experiences.

    c.   Facilitate exploration of alternative coping mechanisms.

    d.   Help identify sources of conflict.

  e. Encourage expression of anxiety, feelings, and concerns.

  f. Focus on personal strengths and skills.

  g. Support a commitment to insight-oriented therapy with an experienced therapist.

D. **Evaluation**

  1. The patient states awareness of stressors precipitating anxiety responses.

  2. The patient reports precipitating stressors absent, reduced, or managed.

  3. Physiologic outcomes: anxiety responses are reduced or eliminated.

  4. Behavioral outcomes: anxiety responses are reduced or eliminated.

  5. Cognitive outcomes: anxiety responses are reduced or eliminated.

  6. Affective outcomes: anxiety responses are reduced or eliminated.

Bibliography

American Psychiatric Association (1987). *Diagnostic and statistical manual of mental disorders (DSM-III-R)* (3rd ed., revised). Washington, DC: Author.

Doenges, M., Townsend, M., & Moorhouse, M. (1988). *Psychiatric care plans: Guidelines for client care*. Philadelphia: F. A. Davis.

Johnson, B. S. (1989). *Psychiatric-mental health nursing: Adaptation and growth* (2nd ed.). Philadelphia: J. B. Lippincott.

Stuart, G., & Sundeen, S. (1987). *Principles and practice of psychiatric nursing* (3rd ed.). St. Louis: C. V. Mosby.

Wilson, H., & Kneisl, C. (1988). *Psychiatric nursing* (3rd ed.). Menlo Park, CA: Addison-Wesley.

STUDY QUESTIONS

1. Which of the following statements best describes Selye's General Adaptation Syndrome?
   a. When stress occurs, the body goes through predictable responses no matter what the stressors are.
   b. When stress occurs, the body's defenses become depleted as they are used.
   c. When stress occurs, the body reacts adversely regardless of the stressors.
   d. When stress occurs, the body becomes less able to deal with subsequent stress.

2. When assessing an anxious patient, the nurse should recognize that a person deals most effectively with stress when at what anxiety level?
   a. mild
   b. moderate
   c. severe
   d. panic

3. Recurring thoughts and behavioral rituals are characteristic of which of the following anxiety disorders?
   a. generalized anxiety disorders
   b. phobias
   c. obsessive-compulsive disorder
   d. dissociative disorder

4. Which group of disorders is characterized by altered identity and recall following a severely stressful experience?
   a. anxiety disorders
   b. dissociative disorders
   c. psychophysiologic disorders
   d. somatization disorders

5. A patient is preoccupied with numerous bodily complaints even after careful diagnostic work reveals no physiologic problems. Which of the following nursing approaches would be therapeutic for this patient?
   a. Listen to the patient's complaints carefully and ask the patient about them frequently.
   b. Acknowledge that the complaints are real to the patient and refocus the patient on other concerns.

   c. Challenge the physical complaints by confronting the patient with the normal diagnostic findings.
   d. Ignore the patient's complaints but have the patient write a list of them.

6. When assessing a patient for recent stressful life events, the nurse should recognize that these refer to changes experienced by the patient that are both:
   a. undesirable and harmful
   b. desirable and growth promoting
   c. positive and negative
   d. unwanted and unhealthy

7. Which of the following nursing approaches would be most therapeutic in assisting a patient to cope with stressful life events?
   a. Encourage the patient to complain about the stresses experienced.
   b. Help the patient to refocus only on the positive aspects of stress.
   c. Avoid thinking about potential future life changes.
   d. Develop ability and patience to deal with life changes.

8. The nurse is teaching a recently diagnosed diabetic patient how to take prescribed insulin. The patient is having difficulty concentrating on what the nurse says. His respirations are becoming shallow and more rapid, and he is beginning to fidget, crossing and uncrossing his legs frequently and picking at his cuticles. His blood sugar level is within normal range. What degree of anxiety is the patient most likely experiencing?
   a. mild
   b. moderate
   c. severe
   d. panic

9. Which initial nursing intervention would be most appropriate for the patient in question 8?
   a. Stop the insulin lesson for awhile, and ask the patient how things are going for him.

b. State that learning about insulin need not be complicated if the patient will just relax.

c. Instruct the patient to pay closer attention to what is being taught because it is vital to his health.

d. Leave the patient for awhile so that he can become more relaxed.

10. After three diabetic teaching sessions, the nurse evaluates that the patient is not progressing well regarding diabetic self-care. In order for the patient to learn, what needs to happen first?
   a. The patient needs to trust himself more.
   b. The patient needs to practice more often.
   c. The patient needs to experience less anxiety.
   d. The patient needs to take control of his illness.

11. Ms. Lant, a newly admitted patient, stays up all night scrubbing the toilet and wash basin and washing her hands over and over. She is constantly bothered by recurrent, intrusive thoughts. Based on this information, the nurse could assume that Ms. Lant suffers from
   a. hypochondriasis
   b. conversion disorder
   c. psychogenic fugue
   d. obsessive-compulsive disorder

12. When implementing nursing care, the nurse should keep in mind that when Ms. Lant's anxiety increases, her ritualistic behaviors likely will
   a. increase
   b. stay the same
   c. decrease
   d. not be related to anxiety

13. Ms. Lant has been on the unit for 3 days. She states that she is feeling more comfortable and at ease on the unit. In light of this change, which nursing intervention could be initiated?
   a. Allow her to engage in her ritualistic behaviors as much as she wants.
   b. Help her think about ways to limit the ritualistic behaviors.
   c. Focus on the ritualistic behaviors every time they occur.
   d. Strictly limit the ritualistic behaviors.

14. Which nursing action should be taken first for a patient exhibiting a higher than usual level of preoperative anxiety?
   a. Ask the patient about his or her perceptions and feelings in relation to the upcoming surgery.
   b. Call to inform the surgeon about the patient's anxiety.
   c. Ask the patient's family to stay with the patient for support.
   d. Teach the patient what he or she needs to know about the upcoming surgery.

ANSWER KEY

1. **Correct response: a**
   Selye found that no matter what kinds of stressors were applied to rats (chemicals, physical, or psychologic stress), their bodies responded with the same types of physiologic changes.
   b. Stress is not necessarily an adverse response.
   c. The body constantly adapts to stress.
   d. Only when stress is overwhelming does the body wear down.
   Comprehension/Physiologic/Assessment

2. **Correct response: a**
   With mild anxiety, the person feels more alert and is able to focus on the problem at hand.
   b. Although the person can still focus and pay attention, with moderate anxiety concentration is reduced.
   c and d. Coping is impaired when anxiety is at severe or panic levels.
   Knowledge/Health Promotion/Assessment

3. **Correct response: c**
   Obsessive-compulsive disorder is characterized by unwanted repetitive thoughts and behaviors. The thoughts are intrusive and the behaviors tend to be concerned with cleanliness, checking, and other rituals.
   a, b, and d. These are other disorders related to anxiety.
   Knowledge/Psychosocial/Analysis

4. **Correct response: b**
   In dissociative disorders, a cluster of recent related events is beyond the recall of the person. These forgotten things can come back into awareness. In one type of dissociative disorder, the person separates his or her emotional self so that he or she feels depersonalized.
   a, c, and d. These are other types of disorders.
   Knowledge/Psychosocial/Analysis (Dx)

5. **Correct response: b**
   After physical factors are ruled out, such somatic complaints are thought to be expressions of anxiety, possibly related to dependency needs. It is important for the nurse to realize that the complaints are real to the patient, but the nurse should not focus on them. Getting the patient to talk about other concerns will encourage expression of anxiety and dependency needs.
   a. Focusing on the somatic symptoms will reinforce them.
   c. Confronting the patient in this manner shows lack of sensitivity to the unconscious nature of the problem and will result in an increase in the patient's anxiety.
   d. Through this action, the nurse merely avoids the problem.
   Application/Safe Care/Implementation

6. **Correct response: c**
   Stressful life events is a concept based on the research of Holmes and Rahe, in which it was found that both positive and negative changes result in stress.
   a, b, and d. None of these responses represents a complete answer to the question asked.
   Knowledge/Psychosocial/Assessment

7. **Correct response: d**
   It takes both ability and patience to adjust to life changes. The greater one's coping skills, the more effectively one can deal with life stresses.
   a, b, and c. These responses are incorrect; the patient needs to look at both positive and negative aspects of change, and also to anticipate potential future changes.
   Application/Health promotion/ Implementation

8. **Correct response: b**
   Moderate anxiety, manifested by rest-

lessness and inability to concentrate, inhibits the learning process.

    a, c, and d. These levels of anxiety have manifestations different from those presented in the scenario.

Comprehension/Physiologic/Assessment

9.   *Correct response: a*

Because the patient's anxiety is increasing, the nurse should stop and assess what is happening. Asking the patient an open-ended question and conveying interest may reduce anxiety and also elicit information on how the patient is dealing with the illness of diabetes. It is important for the nurse to recognize that diabetes constitutes a major life change and is therefore a stressful diagnosis.

    b, c, and d. Through these responses, the nurse avoids having the patient express his concerns.

Analysis/Psychosocial/Implementation

10.   *Correct response: c*

The patient's anxiety must be reduced because it is interfering with his learning.

    a, b, and d. Although all of these interventions are desirable, they cannot be accomplished until the patient's anxiety is reduced.

Application/Safe care/Analysis (Dx)

11.   *Correct response: d*

Obsessive-compulsive disorder is characterized by unwanted recurring thoughts and repetitive, ritualistic behaviors.

    a, b, and c. These responses describe other anxiety-related disorders.

Comprehension/Psychosocial/Analysis (Dx)

12.   *Correct response: a*

Obsessive-compulsive behavior is thought to be an abnormal manifestation of anxiety. If anxiety is increased, the patient likely will increase her ritualistic behaviors, because they serve to alleviate anxiety.

    b, c, and d. These responses would not be expected in obses sive-compulsive disorder.

Analysis/Psychosocial/Implementation

13.   *Correct response: b*

Because compulsive behaviors are used to control anxiety, it is helpful if the patient herself thinks of ways to limit them. This way she stays in control and takes responsibility for her own behaviors.

    a. In this case, the patient stays up all night to do the rituals. While this may be allowed the first few nights, after a trusting relationship has developed, Ms. Lant should be encouraged to modify her behavior.

    c. Focusing on the behaviors will reinforce them.

    d. This would greatly increase Ms. Lant's anxiety, probably leading her to scrub other areas.

Application/Psychosocial/Implementation

14.   *Correct response: a*

The nurse should attempt to assess and reduce the patient's anxiety by listening to the patient, offering support, and correcting any distortions about the upcoming surgery.

    b, c, and d. These interventions could be implemented after talking with the patient.

Application/Safe care/Implementation

Personality Disorders

I. Overview

A. Definitions

1. Personality: early established behavior patterns related to how one thinks, feels, and relates to the environment and to others
2. Personality disorders: various enduring inflexible, maladaptive behavior patterns or traits that may impair functioning and relationships

B. Basic concepts

1. Personality is composed of:
   a. Temperament, largely inherited
   b. Character, largely learned

2. Although a personality disorder may interfere with life situations and relationships, the person usually remains in touch with reality, and entry into the mental health system seldom occurs.
3. Stress typically exacerbates manifestations of personality disorder.
4. Because the person typically has a lack of insight into his or her behavior, effecting behavioral change is unlikely.
5. In severe cases, personality disorder may deteriorate to a psychotic state.

C. Etiology
1. Behavioral patterns to protect the self from threats emerge from early experiences, including:
   a. Early relationships
   b. Actions of others
   c. Material objects
   d. Symbols
2. Defensive behaviors solidify as automatic responses to situations and persons.
3. Rigid responses may develop out of numerous or misperceived threats.
4. Narrow interpretations and the desire to direct or control may evolve.

D. General characteristics of personality disorders
1. Exaggerated, inflexible pattern or traits
2. Restricted or exaggerated moral development
3. Limited or unusual problem-solving skills
4. Impaired communication and interpersonal relationships, relationship conflicts
5. Difficulties in social or occupational situations
6. Defensive behavior against real or perceived threats to self
7. Maintenance of self in mainstream of society despite difficulties
8. Limited or heightened affective responses (ranging from overly sensitive to unemotional or aloof)
9. Lack of insight concerning the unusual components of own behavior; may see others as having problems

II. **Types of personality disorders**
A. Eccentric personality disorders
1. Paranoid disorders: mistaken interpretation of others' motives and actions as threatening to self
2. Schizoid or schizotypal disorder: social detachment with limited expression of emotion, unusual ideas, and peculiar behaviors (schizotypal is more pathologic)

B. Dramatic-erratic personality disorders
1. Borderline personality disorder: instability of mood (with wide ranges of affective responses), relationships, and self-image and identity

    2. Histrionic personality disorder: dramatic, egocentric, attention-seeking response patterns; constant acting or role playing

    3. Narcissistic personality disorder: imbalance in regulating esteem and expression; may have low or high esteem but with expectation of special privileges and consideration

    4. Antisocial (or sociopathic) personality disorder: manipulation and control of others with disregard for social norms; prior to age 18 this may be typified by conduct problems, later it may involve criminal behavior

C. **Anxious or fearful personality disorders**

    1. Avoidant personality disorder: fearfulness of and hypersensitivity to potential rejection or criticism; avoidance of close relationships, but with a dislike of being alone

    2. Dependent personality disorder: dependency, submissiveness to others; passive acceptance of control from more dominant persons

    3. Obsessive-compulsive personality disorder: fear of losing control over situations, objects, and people, with resultant focus on organization, details, responsibilities (see also Chapter 3, Stress, Anxiety, and Anxiety-Related Disorders)

    4. Passive-aggressive personality disorder: indirect expression of anger through passive resistance, delays, argumentativeness

III. **Nursing process in eccentric personality disorders**

    A. **Assessment**

        1. Note characteristic manifestations of paranoid disorders, such as:

            a. Suspiciousness, mistrust

            b. Jealousy

            c. Guardedness

            d. Restricted affect (lack of emotional expression and spontaneous behavior)

            e. Projection (attributing own beliefs and feelings to others)

        2. Assess for manifestations of schizoid or schizotypal disorder, which may include:

            a. Emotional aloofness

            b. Social withdrawal

            c. Oddities of thought, speech, and behavior; peculiar mannerisms, "odd" affect

            d. Detachment (unawareness, neglect of hygiene, social standards, and norms)

        3. Also note other signs of both types of eccentric personality disorders, including:

            a. Impaired social and occupational functioning

            b. Some cognitive impairment

    B. **Analysis and nursing diagnoses**

        1. The nurse should be aware of the patient's fear of closeness and commitment.

      2. Pertinent North American Nursing Diagnosis Association (NANDA) diagnoses could include:
- a. Impaired Verbal Communication
- b. Ineffective Individual Coping
- c. High Risk for Self-Care Deficit
- d. Social Isolation
- e. Altered Thought Processes

C. **Planning and implementation**
1. Take an objective, matter-of-fact approach to patient care.
2. Keep verbal and nonverbal messages clear and consistent.
3. Provide a daily schedule of activities.
4. Maintain focus on reality-based, low-stress topics.
5. Gradually identify feelings implied or expressed by the patient.
6. Gradually involve the patient in group situations.

D. **Evaluation**
1. Little change in behavior may be seen.
2. Some improvement may be seen, marked by such milestones as:
   - a. Attachment with one or two people
   - b. Ability to function in social and occupational situations for extended periods
   - c. Reduction in sharing bizarre or paranoid ideas with others
   - d. Some attempt to control or reduce unusual mannerisms or affects

IV. **Nursing process in dramatic-erratic personality disorders**
    A. Assessment
1. Note characteristic manifestations of borderline personality disorder, such as:
   - a. Intense affect
   - b. Extreme emotional lability
   - c. Impulsiveness
   - d. Unstable, conflictual relationships
   - e. Controlling, manipulative behavior
   - f. Feelings of emptiness and isolation
   - g. Self-destructive behavior
2. Observe for common manifestations of histrionic personality disorder, including:
   - a. Dramatic, overemphasized behavior
   - b. Exaggerated emotions, temper tantrums
   - c. Difficulty and lack of commitment in relationships
   - d. Overtones of sexuality, sexual expression, and flamboyance
   - e. Impressionability
   - f. Dependence on authority figures
3. Narcissistic personality disorder may present with:
   - a. Grandiose thinking
   - b. Exaggerated sense of self-importance

       c.   Excessive drive for success and power
       d.   Attention-seeking behavior
       e.   Rationalization for failures
       f.   Difficulty sustaining relationships
       g.   Some degree of sexual confusion, possible promiscuity or homosexuality

4. Assess for common features of antisocial personality disorder, including:
    a. Manipulative, controlling behavior
    b. Extroverted, charming manner
    c. Interference with others' rights
    d. Impaired conscience, with lying, cheating, conning, possible criminal behaviors
    e. Desire for immediate pleasure and needs gratification
    f. Lack of concern about right and wrong, socially accepted morals and values
    g. Lack of commitment and intimacy in relationships
    h. Poor work history

B. Analysis and nursing diagnoses
1. The nurse needs to rule out major thought or affective disorders.
2. The nurse also needs to keep in mind that these patients commonly have poor self-esteem, despite their apparent egocentricity.
3. Pertinent NANDA diagnoses may include:
    a. Ineffective Individual Coping
    b. High Risk for Injury
    c. Disturbance in Self-Concept: Personal Identity
    d. High Risk for Violence

C. Planning and implementation
1. Take a concerned, matter-of-fact, consistent approach.
2. Be alert for manipulation (e.g., flattery, flirting, verbal attacks).
3. Give feedback to confront inappropriate behavior.
4. Examine consequences of appropriate and inappropriate responses or behavior.
5. Avoid rescuing or rejecting; deal with manipulation and immediate needs vs. delayable needs.
6. Set limits on manipulation and disregard for rights of others.
7. Give positive reinforcement for achievement of goals.
8. Explore the patient's feelings; examine constructive means of expressing anger.
9. Use problem-solving approaches to help the patient explore changes.

D. Evaluation
1. Little change in behavior may be seen.
2. Some improvement may be seen, as manifested by:

a. Reduced anxiety and intense acting-out
b. Reduced aggression toward self and others
c. Increased impulse control
d. Decreased manipulation
e. Adherence to rules, particularly in structured environments and relationships

V. Nursing process in anxious or fearful personality disorders

A. Assessment

1. Observe for features of avoidant personality disorder, such as:
   a. Hypersensitivity to others' reactions and criticisms
   b. Fear of rejection or failure
   c. Desire for affection and attention (but socially withdrawn because of fear)
   d. Fear or discomfort associated with being alone
   e. Overly serious, blunted emotional expression
   f. Devaluation of personal abilities and achievements

2. Assess for dependent personality disorder, which may be marked by:
   a. Lack of self-confidence, poor self-esteem
   b. Indecisiveness
   c. Difficulty with independent behavior
   d. Clinging, reliant behavior
   e. Submissive behavior
   f. Devaluation of personal abilities and achievements

3. Evaluate for manifestations of obsessive-compulsive personality disorder, which may include:
   a. Relentless striving for organization and order
   b. Controlling, demanding behavior
   c. Excessive dedication to work
   d. Perfectionism, overattention to detail
   e. Rigidity
   f. Moralistic, judgmental attitude toward others
   g. Indirect expressions of anger

4. Note signs of passive-aggressive personality disorder, such as:
   a. Indirect expression of anger
   b. Procrastination, forgetfulness
   c. Protests about unrealistic demands and expectations of others
   d. Expressions of resentment and pouty, irritable behavior when required to perform an undesirable task
   e. Possible unreasonable criticism or judgment of authority figures

B. Nursing diagnoses

1. Ineffective Individual Coping
2. Self-Concept Disturbance

3. Social Isolation
C. **Planning and implementation**

1. Establish a caring, consistent therapeutic relationship.
2. Gently give feedback to confront inappropriate, nonproductive, unsatisfying behaviors.
3. Encourage the patient to discuss feelings of fear and anger behind his or her behavior.
4. Encourage the patient to verbalize feelings of fear, rejection, inferiority, anger.
5. Avoid argument or debate; use humor and provide gentle feedback.
6. Establish clear expectations for behavior, responsibility, achievement.
7. Support practice with decision making and assertiveness.
8. Facilitate successful experiences with task completion and goal achievement.

D. **Evaluation**
1. Little change in behavior may be seen.
2. Some improvement may be seen, as marked by:
   a. Some degree of awareness of own behavior and effect on others
   b. Some modification of behavior patterns

Bibliography

American Psychiatric Association (1987). *Diagnostic and statistical manual of mental disorders (DSM-III-R)* (3rd ed., revised). Washington, DC: Author.

Johnson, B. S. (1989). *Psychiatric-mental health nursing: Adaptation and growth* (2nd ed.). Philadelphia: J. B. Lippincott.

Stuart, G. W., & Sundeen, S. J. (1987). *Principles and practice of psychiatric nursing* (3rd ed.). St. Louis: C. V. Mosby.

Wilson, H. S., & Kneisl, C. R. (1988). *Psychiatric nursing* (3rd ed.). Menlo Park, CA: Addison-Wesley.

STUDY QUESTIONS

1. Mrs. Jones has a dependent personality disorder. She has been submissive to her husband's wishes and has taken direction for their lives from him for 25 years. Recently, Mr. Jones died. The nurse would expect Mrs. Jones to experience which of the following responses?
   a. relief, following grief, to begin to live her life in independent ways
   b. increase in dependent and passive symptoms
   c. take-charge and decisive attitude during this crisis period
   d. paranoia about relationships

2. Which of the following is characteristic of the histrionic personality disorder?
   a. very focused on detail
   b. limited expression of emotion
   c. dramatic, always "on stage"
   d. disregard for social norms

3. Mr. Marks, aged 24, has been diagnosed with schizoid personality disorder. Which of the following behaviors would the nurse *not* likely see during assessment?
   a. social detachment
   b. limited emotional expression
   c. bizarre ideas and mannerisms
   d. focused attention on self in relationships

4. Mr. Brown, aged 36, has an anxious personality type. He lacks confidence and seems to reject others in relationships before he can be rejected. He sometimes has difficulty accomplishing work assignments efficiently or well because he is afraid of failing. Which of the following nursing diagnoses would be most appropriate for Mr. Brown?
   a. Disturbance in Self-Concept: Personal Identity
   b. Altered Thought Processes
   c. Self-Care Deficit
   d. High Risk for Violence: Self-Directed

5. Which of the following statements regarding persons with personality disorders is true?
   a. They typically maintain themselves in the mainstream of society.
   b. They often become psychotic when their illness becomes more acute.
   c. They commonly seek psychotherapy.
   d. Prognosis for recovery with therapy is good.

6. Mrs. Wright, aged 48, describes herself as a "very religious person" with strong opinions on "what is right and what is wrong." She is quite judgmental regarding others' beliefs and life-styles. Which of the following principles could support evaluation of Mrs. Wright's behavior as a personality disorder?
   a. Religious fanatics almost always have personality disorders.
   b. Restricted or exaggerated moral development may be a symptom.
   c. Flexible belief systems raise doubts about mental stability.
   d. Judgmental behavior, including self-insight, is typical of personality disorders.

7. Mr. Joe, aged 47, has been renting a room from Mrs. White, aged 67, to whom he acts attentive and charming. He is sometimes late with his rent, but he always seems to have a good reason, and "he is such a nice man" that Mrs. White is not persistent in collecting from him. She even loans him money one day to help "meet expenses for his sick mother." She is quite surprised to find his things gone, with no explanation or warning, at the end of the month. Based on this information, Mr. Joe may well have which of the following personality disorders?
   a. Obsessive-compulsive disorder
   b. Paranoid disorder
   c. Avoidant disorder
   d. Antisocial disorder

8. Mr. Allen, aged 43, is perfectionistic, very particular about following rules, and focused on details. He is quite dedi-

cated to his job and effective in producing work, but he always insists on doing things his way. Analysis of his rigidity likely would reveal

a. fear of loss of control
b. fear of rejection
c. fear of goal achievement
d. fear of attention

9. Ms. Elena, aged 29, has a history of conflictual relationships. She expresses the desire for friends but acts in alienating ways with people who befriend her. Which of the following would be an important nursing intervention for Ms. Elena?

a. Help her find friends who are patient and extra caring.
b. Establish a therapeutic relationship in which role-modeling and role-playing may occur.
c. Realize that she cannot change, and accept her as she is.
d. Point out her difficulties in relationships and suggest areas for improvement.

10. Ms. Rose, aged 59, has a history of problems with people and job positions. She is inflexible, opinionated, and defensive. However, she complains to the nurse that "people are so hard to get along with" and "if people weren't so stupid and lazy, things would go much more smoothly." Why is this behavior fairly typical of a person with a personality disorder?

a. Personality disorders are most common in women with relationship problems.
b. Lack of insight and blaming others are characteristic behaviors in personality disorders.
c. Loud, opinionated behavior is typical in personality disorders.
d. Rationalization and identification are major coping measures in personality disorders.

11. Persons with antisocial personality disorders come to the attention of social agencies more frequently than do persons with other personality disorders because

a. They are charming and sincere in relationships.
b. They are more likely to seek therapy.
c. They are often engaged in criminal activity.
d. They are most likely to become psychotic and be hospitalized.

12. Ms. Pai, aged 39, has a schizotypal personality disorder manifested by limited social skills, bizarre thoughts and mannerisms, and inability to hold a job. She has few relatives (none of whom will accept her), and she is currently living on the streets with other homeless persons. Tonight, she is brought into the emergency room by the police, who found her wandering in the street. Nursing assessment reveals a high fever and a badly infected leg. After infection is controlled, a priority nursing diagnosis would be

a. Altered Role Performance
b. Diversional Activity Deficit
c. High Risk for Violence: Self-Directed
d. Ineffective Individual Coping

13. Mr. Smith, aged 41, thinks people talk about him behind his back and are out to get his job. Hypersensitive to criticism, he often believes his actions are misjudged. He is mistrustful and jealous in relationships. Which of the following coping measures is Mr. Smith exhibiting in his paranoid behavior patterns?

a. projection
b. introjection
c. displacement
d. sublimation

14. Some patients with personality disorders are defensive and emotionally labile and may become suddenly and explosively angry. When interacting with such a patient, the nurse should

a. Point out how angry he is becoming; confront the angry behavior.
b. Use gentle and caring touch to calm the patient.

c. Tell the patient to calm down and stop using derogatory language.
d. Take a calm, quiet, nonconfrontational approach; do not argue.

15. Which of the following is the best definition of personality disorder?
   a. a false belief that resists modification
   b. a mental state in which the person's ability to perceive reality is impaired
   c. an inflexible behavior pattern that causes problems in functioning and relationships
   d. a mental disorder involving psychotic disturbances in thought association and affect

16. Ms. Violet, aged 18, is very self-involved and believes she is entitled to special privileges in her community; as she puts it, "After all, my family has lived here for over 100 years." She seems preoccupied with issues of societal position and wealth. She treats others somewhat like servants and is insensitive to their needs or reactions. Which of the following personality disorders most likely would apply to Ms. Violet?
   a. narcissistic disorder
   b. histrionic disorder
   c. antisocial disorder
   d. avoidance disorder

ANSWER KEY

1. **Correct response: b**
Stress increases symptoms in personality disorders.
   a and c. These indicate a change in an ingrained personality pattern.
   d. This is another personality disorder behavior.
Application/Psychosocial/Assessment

2. **Correct response: c**
The histrionic personality is dramatic, reactive, and attention-seeking.
   a. This describes obsessive-compulsive disorder.
   b. This describes paranoid and schizoid personality disorders.
   d. This describes antisocial personality disorder.
Knowledge/Psychosocial/Assessment

3. **Correct response: d**
A schizoid personality is detached, aloof, and socially isolated rather than attention-seeking.
   a, b, and c. These behaviors are characteristic of a schizoid personality disorder.
Knowledge/Psychosocial/Assessment

4. **Correct response: a**
The anxious-fearful personality has problems with insecurity and esteem.
   b and c. These persons do not have major thought disturbances or self-care problems.
   d. There are no data to support suicide potential.
Application/Safe care/Analysis (Dx)

5. **Correct response: a**
Persons with personality disorders typically are functional with inflexible personality patterns.
   b. These persons are not usually psychotic.
   c. These persons typically do not seek treatment.
   d. These persons commonly have poor prognoses because of lack of insight and unwillingness to seek therapy.
Comprehension/Psychosocial/Assessment

6. **Correct response: b**
Absence of moral values or rigid adherence to moral values is characteristic.
   a. Religious fanatics may be motivated by other psychodynamics (e.g., psychotic states).
   c. Flexible belief systems may indicate health.
   d. Insight usually is lacking.
Application/Psychosocial/Analysis (Dx)

7. **Correct response: d**
Mr. Joe's behavior is typical of the antisocial personality.
   a, b, and c. The charming behavior lacking in social accountability is not characteristic of these disorders.
Analysis/Psychosocial/Analysis (Dx)

8. **Correct response: a**
Persons with obsessive-compulsive disorder have problems with loss of control.
   b, c, and d. These features are more characteristic of other personality disorders.
Application/Psychosocial/Analysis (Dx)

9. **Correct response: b**
Starting with a therapeutic one-to-one relationship is important in attempting to modify Ms. Elena's behavior.
   a, c, and d. These interventions would not assist Ms. Elena, initially, in learning new patterns of relating.
Analysis/Safe care/Implementation

10. **Correct response: b**
Lack of self-insight is a major characteristic.
   a and d. These are incorrect statements.
   c. This is not typical of all personality disorders.
Analysis/Psychosocial/Analysis (Dx)

11. **Correct response: c**
Persons with antisocial personality disorder lack social accountability and moral

values and may engage in criminal activities.

    a. Although this may seem true, it does not increase frequency of contact with social agencies.

    b and d. These are incorrect statements.

Comprehension/Psychosocial/Analysis (Dx)]

12. *Correct response: d*

    Ineffective coping is well supported by the data.

    a, b, and c. These are not well supported, nor very pertinent.

Application/Safe care/Analysis (Dx)

13. *Correct response: a*

    A major defense mechanism in paranoid behavior is projection of one's own fears, emotions, or desires on others.

    b, c, and d. These are not pertinent defenses.

Application/Psychosocial/Analysis (Dx)

14. *Correct response: d*

    An important intervention with angry behavior is a calm, nonconfrontational, nonargumentative manner.

    a, b, and c. These approaches could exacerbate anger and trigger explosive behavior.

Analysis/Safe care/Planning

15. *Correct response: c*

    a, b, and d. These responses describe delusion, psychosis, and schizophrenia, respectively.

Comprehension/Psychosocial/NA

16. *Correct response: a*

    Ms. Violet's behavior is self-absorbed and "entitled" and supports narcissistic behavior.

    b, c, and d. None of these disorders is supported by this patient's behavior patterns.

Application/Psychosocial/Analysis (Dx)

Affective Disorders and Suicidal Behavior

I. Overview

A. Definitions

1. Affective disorders: a group of disorders involving disturbances of mood, or emotional and behavioral response patterns ranging from elation or agitation to extreme sadness, emotional isolation, and immobility. Types include:
   a. Depressive disorders
   b. Bipolar (manic-depressive) disorders
2. Suicidal behavior: thoughts or acts involving taking one's own life, including:
   a. Suicidal threat: a specific reference to suicidal intent, usually accompanied by behavioral changes

      b.   Suicidal gesture: a self-destructive act that does not cause serious injury but attracts attention or concern; may be followed by more serious attempt

      c.   Suicidal attempt: a self-destructive act that has the potential outcome of death

B. **Basic concepts**

1. Ranges in emotion are part of the human condition.
2. Grief is a "normal" powerful emotional state following loss.
3. Maladaptive responses to emotional issues involve suppression of feelings or overelaboration of intense feelings.
4. Particular risk factors for affective disorders include:
   a. Family history
   b. Childhood experiences in hostile, negative environment
   c. Lack of intimate, confiding relationship
   d. Medical illness
   e. Giving birth within the past 6 months
5. A suicidal person often wants to live but can think of no other alternative to relieve or resolve the intolerable pain or multiple problems that he or she is experiencing.
6. Suicide rarely is spontaneous; usually it results from years of defeat and reduced coping ability.
7. The person almost always gives verbal or behavioral clues of suicidal intent.
8. About 65% of persons who attempt suicide signal intent to a health care provider sometime during the 6-month period before the attempt.
9. Suicidal behavior may be a form of communication between the suicidal person and significant other(s).
10. Suicidal persons generally are not psychotic.
11. Suicidal behavior occurs in all ethnic, racial, and socioeconomic groups.
12. Although women attempt suicide more frequently, men are more often successful.
13. Incidence of suicidal behavior peaks between ages 45 and 54 in women and steadily increases with age in men.
14. Incidence is lower in married adults and higher in divorced or widowed adults.
15. Incidence is increasing in adolescents.
16. Statistically, suicide is the 10th or 11th cause of death in the United States (counting reported suicides only).

C. **Etiology**

1. Possible biochemical or genetic factors associated with affective disorders include:
   a. Alteration in biogenic amines, neurotransmitters consisting of catecholamines and indolamines (e.g., serotonin)

    b. Electrolyte disturbance: increased cortisol and sodium re-tention

    c. Genetic: possible genetic predisposition, especially in bipo-lar disorders

2. Psychoanalytic factors (Freud's theory) include:

    a. Internalization of angry and aggressive feelings that should be directed to an ambivalent loved object or person

    b. Feelings of self-anger and aggression leading to negative ideations about self

3. Ego-psychologic factors (Bibring's theory) include:

    a. Real or imagined loss of an important object

    b. Inability to obtain object, with resultant feelings of help-lessness, hostility, and reduced self-esteem

4. Cognitive factors (Beck's theory) include:

    a. Negative cognitions (unchallenged errors in thinking) of self, of the world, and of the future—a cognitive trial (Table 5–1)

    b. Negative cognitions of self: perception of self as unattrac-tive, deprived, defeated, deserted, incompetent in all areas of life

    c. Negative cognitions of the world: perception of the world as demanding and unyielding

    d. Negative cognitions of the future: perception of the future as involving nothing but failure

5. The original learned helplessness model (Seligman's theory) ex-plained the relationship between loss of control over one's envi-ronment and one's consequent feelings of helplessness, power-lessness, and depression. This model did not address decreased self-esteem, chronicity, and generality of helplessness, however. The addition of the attribution theory, which states that people give themselves explanations of why events occur as they do, re-solved this problem. These explanations include:

    a. Internal vs. external explanation: The event occurred as it did because of self vs. situation; impacts on self-esteem.

    b. Stable vs. unstable explanation: The event occurred as it did because of causes that are long-term and that will per-sist vs. causes that are transient or short-term; impacts on the chronicity of helplessness.

    c. Global vs. specific explanation: The event occurred as it did because the cause is pervasive and will be influential in many settings vs. the cause is limited to a specific event or concern; impacts on the generality of helplessness.

    d. A depressed person has an idiosyncratic way of explaining negative occurrences in terms of internal, stable, and global attributions.

TABLE 5-1.
Common Negative Cognitions

NEGATIVE COGNITION	DESCRIPTION	EXAMPLE
Overgeneralization	The belief that everything will go wrong because of a single negative occurrence; the act of blowing things out of proportion. Key words indicative of overgeneralization include "never" and "always."	After making a low grade in algebra, the student says, "I will never learn this stuff."
All-or-nothing thinking	Viewing everything in extremes—either black or white, with no middle ground	John takes pictures at his friends wedding. All but three of the pictures were perfect. John was dissatisfied because all the pictures were not perfect and considered himself to be a failure at photography.
Should statements	Using "should," "shouldn't," "must," and "ought to" statements to establish standards for self and others. Should statements in general lead to frustration. Those directed toward oneself lead to guilt; those directed at others lead to anger and resentment.	John (from previous example) said to himself, "I should have done all of them right." A student told herself that she ought to be able to read 300 pages of her nursing text per night with complete comprehension.
Labeling	Applying negatively loaded labels to oneself or others	After the student in the previous example was unable to comprehend the 300 pages of her nursing text, she said, "I'm a dumb idiot."
Mindreading	Jumping to conclusions regarding another person's reactions without checking out those reactions with the other person	You're having an enjoyable lunch with a friend, but the friend looks dejected. You ask what the problem is. After coaxing, he says, "I know you think that I'm a bad person."
Fortune telling	Being absolutely convinced that things will not turn out right, no matter what the evidence to the contrary	You are to meet your partner's parents for the first time. You tell your partner that you know that this is a mistake, that this meeting will be a complete disaster. Your partner tries to reassure you, but you know better.

6. Life stressors may serve as precipitating factors; examples include:
   a. Experienced or perceived losses
   b. Life changes
   c. Role conflicts
   d. Reduced financial or social support
7. The integrative factors model posits that neither biochemical or genetic factors nor psychosocial or environmental factors adequately explain the etiology of depressive disorders. Rather, depression is viewed as an interaction of various biochemical, experiential, and behavioral factors.

      8.   Physical factors associated with suicidal behavior may include:
          a.   Illness, especially life-threatening, long-term, or disfiguring
          b.   Isolation
          c.   Biochemical factors associated with depression
      9.   Psychosocial factors may include:
          a.   Recent loss, grief, depression
          b.   Numerous life stressors
          c.   Lacking or limited resources, interpersonal supports
          d.   Alcoholism, drug abuse
          e.   Lack of effective communication, feelings of emotional isolation
          f.   History of suicide attempts; formulated suicide plan
     10.   Statistical predictors of high risk include age, sex, race, and marital status.

II. Types of affective disorders
A. Depressive disorders
      1.   Major depression, single episode: one-time occurrence of major sadness or depression
      2.   Major depression, recurrent: repeated episodes of major sadness or depression separated by long intervals, occurring in clusters or increasing with age
      3.   Dysthymia: chronic depressive mood problems occurring in the absence of a major depressive episode or organic or psychotic diagnosis
B. Bipolar disorders
      1.   Bipolar, mixed: rapid intermingling of depressed and manic behavior
      2.   Bipolar, manic: most recent or current episode displaying overactive, agitated behavior
      3.   Bipolar, depressed: most recent or current behavior displaying major depression
      4.   Cyclothymia: numerous occurrences of abnormally elevated or irritable moods and abnormally depressed moods over a period of at least 2 years
C. Suicidal behavior
      1.   Indirect self-destructive behavior: usually long-term, potentially life-threatening (e.g., alcoholism, heroin addiction)
      2.   Direct self-destructive behavior: has intent of the outcome of death; the person is aware of the desired outcome

III. Nursing process in depressive disorders
A. Assessment
      1.   Observe for physiologic responses, which may include:
          a.   Altered appetite (increased or decreased)
          b.   Altered sleep pattern (insomnia, hypersomnia)
          c.   Constipation
          d.   Easy fatigability

   e. Somatic complaints of aches and pains
   f. Weight change (increased or decreased)
   g. Indigestion
   h. Restless, undirected activity
  2. Note any characteristic behavioral responses, such as:
   a. Psychomotor retardation (e.g., walking and talking slowly)
   b. Decreased motivation
   c. Anhedonia—loss of interest in once-pleasurable activities (e.g., sex, work, social interaction) leading to impaired functioning
   d. Crying spells
   e. Frequent demands and complaints
   f. Lack of spontaneity
   g. Poor personal hygiene and grooming
   h. Isolation, withdrawal
   i. Lack of energy
   j. Passive-aggressive behavior
   k. Suicide attempt(s)
  3. Note cognitive responses, which may include:
   a. Indecisiveness
   b. Reduced concentration and attention span
   c. Negative thoughts about self, the world, and the future
   d. Constant rumination
   e. Somatic delusions
   f. Poverty of ideas
  4. Assess for characteristic affective responses, such as:
   a. Sadness, despondency
   b. Anger, agitation, resentfulness
   c. Anxiety, guilt, decreased self-esteem
   d. Hopelessness, helplessness
   e. Loneliness
   f. Worthlessness
   g. Apathy
B. **Nursing diagnoses**
  1. Ineffective Individual Coping
  2. Altered Nutrition: Less Than or More Than Body Requirements
  3. Self-Care Deficit: Hygiene, Grooming, Feeding
  4. Disturbance in Self-Concept: Self-Esteem
  5. Sleep Pattern Disturbance
  6. Impaired Social Interaction
C. **Planning and implementation**
  1. Facilitate adequate nutrition (e.g., provide smaller or larger portions, consider food preferences, stay with the patient during meals).
  2. Assist the patient in developing a daily schedule that balances activity and rest.

3. Promote sleep with daily exercise and activities and bedtime relaxation interventions (e.g., quiet time, back rubs, music).
4. Assist with hygiene and grooming as needed.
5. Have brief, therapeutic interactions with the patient.
6. Don't force conversation, but encourage participation in social interaction and activity.
7. Assist the patient to identify feelings and reduce negative cognitions (see Table 5–1).
8. Institute suicide precautions as necessary.
9. Facilitate successful problem solving and reinforcement by structuring simple, manageable tasks.
10. Administer antidepressant medications, as ordered.

D. Evaluation

1. The patient exhibits improved coping skills.
2. The patient maintains adequate nutritional status.
3. The patient demonstrates improved self-care ability.
4. The patient reports and displays improved self-concept and increased self-esteem.
5. The patient exhibits improved sleep patterns.
6. The patient maintains social interaction to the extent possible.

IV. Nursing process in bipolar disorders

A. Assessment

1. Evaluate for common physiologic responses in bipolar disorders, which may include:
   a. Reduced appetite due to hyperactivity
   b. Physical exhaustion due to hyperactivity
   c. Delirium and stupor
   d. Insomnia
2. Note characteristic behavioral responses, such as:
   a. Demanding behavior, insensitivity
   b. Impulsiveness, lack of inhibition
   c. Manipulative, domineering approach
   d. Narcissism
   e. Low tolerance for frustration
   f. Oversensitivity to criticism
   g. Inappropriate singing, dancing, laughing, joking
   h. Boisterousness, loudness
   i. Talkativeness, push of speech
   j. Hyperactivity (talking and moving quickly), restlessness, excessive energy
   k. Hypersexuality
   l. Spending sprees
   m. Inability to carry out tasks
   n. Engagement in high-risk behavior (e.g., reckless driving, substance abuse, indiscriminate sexual activity)

3. Assess for typical cognitive responses, including:
   a. Grandiose and persecutory delusions
   b. Flight of ideas
   c. Short attention span, poor concentration, poor retention and recall, easy distractibility
   d. Disorientation
   e. Poor insight
   f. Impaired judgment
   g. Tangential thought
4. Note affective responses, such as:
   a. Emotional lability, with mood swings from cheerfulness, euphoria, elation, and exultation to sadness, depression, and even irritability, anger, or rage
   b. Fluctuating sense of self-worth and self-confidence

B. **Nursing diagnoses**
   1. Constipation
   2. Ineffective Individual Coping
   3. High Risk for Injury
   4. Altered Nutrition: Less Than Body Requirements
   5. Self-Care Deficit: Hygiene, Grooming, Feeding
   6. Sleep Pattern Disturbance
   7. Altered Thought Processes

C. **Planning and implementation**
   1. Promote adequate nutrition (e.g., offer the patient high-calorie foods that can be eaten "on the run"; stay with the patient during meals).
   2. Reduce stimulation throughout the day, especially before bedtime.
   3. Promote rest periods; enhance relaxation (e.g., reduce noise, promote quiet time).
   4. Assist with self-care as necessary.
   5. Promote bowel regularity through adequate dietary roughage, adequate fluid intake, and establishment of a regular schedule for defecation.
   6. Take a matter-of-fact and consistent approach in describing acceptable behavior and realistic limits.
   7. Provide the patient with simple tasks that focus attention and yield successful completion.
   8. Assist the patient to think through consequences of behavior and to control his behavior.
   9. Provide a safe environment and patient monitoring to reduce the risk of accidents and injury.
   10. Administer lithium, as ordered.

D. **Evaluation**
   1. The patient maintains good bowel elimination patterns.

    2. The patient exhibits improved coping skills.

    3. The patient remains injury-free.

    4. The patient maintains adequate nutritional status.

    5. The patient demonstrates improved self-care ability.

    6. The patient exhibits improved sleep patterns.

    7. The patient demonstrates improved cognition.

V. Nursing process in suicidal behavior

A. Assessment

    1. Observe for physiologic responses suggestive of suicidal behavior, such as:

       a. Altered appetite

       b. Altered sleep pattern

       c. Somatic complaints, illness

       d. Easy fatigability

    2. Note any uncharacteristic behavioral responses, such as:

       a. Engagement in potentially self-destructive activities and life patterns

       b. Psychomotor retardation

       c. Decreased motivation, anhedonia

       d. Withdrawal from activities and relationships

       e. Verbalizations concerning giving up and ending life; expression of suicidal intent or plan

       f. Giving away of valued possessions, assessment of financial value after death

       g. Suicide gestures, attempts

    3. Assess for such cognitive responses as:

       a. Reduced concentration and attention span

       b. Negative cognitions about self, life, future

       c. Rumination concerning losses and stresses or verbal withdrawal

       d. Poor decision making, impaired judgment

    4. Note altered affective responses, such as:

       a. Sadness, despondency

       b. Anger, resentfulness

       c. Anxiety, guilt, self-disgust

       d. Hopelessness, helplessness

       e. Loneliness ("no one cares")

       f. Worthlessness ("I'm no good")

       g. Apathy

B. Nursing diagnoses

    1. Ineffective Family Coping

    2. Ineffective Individual Coping

    3. Grieving, Dysfunctional

    4. Hopelessness

    5. Powerlessness

6. Disturbance in Self-Concept: Self-Esteem or Personal Identity
7. High Risk for Violence: Self-Directed

C. **Planning and implementation**
1. Evaluate the patient's degree of risk, noting:
   a. Warning signs
   b. Intent to harm self (Note: Asking about intent does not increase the likelihood of suicidal behavior.)
   c. Concreteness of suicide plan
   d. Available resources
2. Determine the presence of high-risk factors.
3. Determine the degree of resources, support systems.
4. Take warning signs seriously.
5. Remove dangerous and potentially lethal materials or objects when possible.
6. Place the patient in a safe, protective environment and monitor closely and consistently—or mobilize support.
7. Establish a firm but supportive relationship.
8. Encourage the patient to talk about stressors; feelings of pain, anger, and anguish; and suicide plans.
9. Listen empathically.
10. Communicate your presence and desire to protect the patient from harming himself or herself.
11. Be aware that suicide risk increases as depression improves.
12. Reinforce the patient's desire to resolve problems, to live.
13. Assist the patient with problem solving; break problems down to more manageable parts.
14. Teach family members about warning signs and encourage them to provide support.
15. Refer the patient for outpatient treatment.

D. **Evaluation**
1. The patient exhibits improved coping skills.
2. Family members also demonstrate improved coping.
3. The family reports and exhibits functional grieving processes.
4. The patient reports decreased feelings of hopelessness and powerlessness.
5. The patient reports and demonstrates improved self-concept, with increased self-esteem and better sense of personal identity.
6. The patient refrains from attempts at self-harm.

Bibliography

American Psychiatric Association (1987). *Diagnostic and statistical manual of mental disorders (DSM-III-R)* (3rd ed., revised). Washington, DC: Author.

Johnson, B. S. (1989). *Psychiatric-mental health nursing: Adaptation and growth* (2nd ed.). Philadelphia: J. B. Lippincott.

Stuart, G. W., & Sundeen, S. J. (1987). *Principles and practice of psychiatric nursing* (3rd ed.). St. Louis: C. V. Mosby.

Wilson, H. S., & Kneisl, C. R. (1988). *Psychiatric nursing* (3rd ed.). Menlo Park, CA: Addison-Wesley.

STUDY QUESTIONS

1. In what ways are bipolar disorder and major depression alike?
   a. Both are disturbances in thinking.
   b. Both have strong genetic underpinnings.
   c. Both are mood disorders.
   d. Both are equally common in men and women.
2. Neurotransmitters speculated to be involved in the etiology of affective disorders include
   a. decreased norepinephrine and serotonin in depressive disorder
   b. decreased norepinephrine and increased serotonin in depressive disorder
   c. increased serotonin and norepinephrine in bipolar disorder
   d. increased serotonin and decreased norepinephrine in bipolar disorder
3. Which model of depression addresses the issues of negative ideations about self, world, and the future?
   a. psychoanalytic model
   b. cognitive model
   c. learned helplessness model
   d. integrative model
4. Bipolar disorder is characterized by
   a. a series of recurrent depressive episodes
   b. two depressive episodes
   c. manic episodes that may be followed by a depressive episode
   d. a depressive episode followed by dysthymia
5. A patient states that she isn't doing well in her English class because she only made a "B" on her term paper, and she thought she ought to have made an "A." Which negative cognitions is this patient demonstrating?
   a. mind-reading and overgeneralization
   b. overgeneralization and fortune telling
   c. labeling and all-or-nothing thinking
   d. all-or-nothing thinking and should statements
6. After talking with Mr. Johns, who is hospitalized for depression, the nurse concludes that his explanations of his situation are consistent with the learned helplessness model reformulated. His explanations are, therefore
   a. internal, unstable, and global
   b. external, unstable, and specific
   c. internal, stable, and global
   d. external, stable, and specific
7. Mr. Johns implies that things will always be bad for him, at all times and in all situations. The nurse recognizes that this type of thinking is an example of
   a. unstable and global explanations and all-or-nothing thinking
   b. stable and global explanations and overgeneralization
   c. stable and global explanations and all-or-nothing thinking
   d. unstable and specific explanations and overgeneralization
8. A patient displaying manic behavior likely would exhibit which of the following symptoms?
   a. excessive spending, poverty of ideas, impulsiveness, and exultation
   b. hypersexuality, apathy, poor insight, and irritability
   c. low tolerance for frustration, lack of inhibition, push of speech, and social isolation
   d. labile affects, flight of ideas, clang association, and impaired judgment
9. Mr. James has a diagnosis of bipolar disorder, manic type. He is very hyperactive and has not slept in 4 days. Which of the following nursing interventions would be most appropriate for Mr. James?
   a. encouraging the physician to prescribe restraints
   b. reducing distractions and encouraging brief periods of rest
   c. observing the patient in the hope that he will settle down soon
   d. isolating the patient in his room until he calms down

10. Mr. James is creating considerable chaos on the ward by his dominating and manipulative behavior. Which of the following nursing interventions would best deal with this behavior?
    a. Provide the patient with alternative behaviors.
    b. Tell the patient that his behavior is unacceptable.
    c. Work with the treatment team to exert ward control.
    d. Establish specific limits on behavior.

11. Ms. Small was admitted to the psychiatric ward from the medical intensive care unit after receiving treatment for a deliberate overdose of prescribed antidepressant medication. The nurse caring for Ms. Small should be aware that warning signs for suicide include
    a. detailed plans and auditory hallucination
    b. availability of method and neologisms
    c. feelings of hopelessness and previous suicide attempts
    d. abrupt behavioral changes and narcissism

12. Recognizing the dynamics of suicide, which of the following nursing actions would be most appropriate for Ms. Small?
    a. Let her spend time alone to reflect on her suicide attempt.
    b. Encourage her to verbalize her feelings and pain.

c. Give her a brief account of the current events to bring her up to date.
d. Avoid the topic of suicide.

13. Ms. Small tells the nurse that her boyfriend ended their relationship and that she would "rather be dead than live without him." Based on this information, the nurse's short-term plan should include which of the following goals?
    a. Ms. Small will find another boyfriend.
    b. Ms. Small will recognize that she was too dependent on this boyfriend.
    c. Ms. Small will develop adaptive dating skills.
    d. Ms. Small will state that she feels okay being alive.

14. Mr. and Mrs. Ball come to the outpatient clinic. Mrs. Ball says that she is concerned about her husband because she never knows what to expect of him; he's sometimes happy and sometimes sad. Sometimes he displays self-confidence while at other times he is extremely down on himself. During assessment, which information should the nurse gather first?
    a. information about Mr. Ball's symptoms, their impact and duration
    b. information about Mr. and Mrs. Ball's marital relationship
    c. information about psychopathology in Mr. Ball's family
    d. information about Mr. Ball's academic achievement.

ANSWER KEY

1. **Correct response: c**
   Both bipolar disorder and major depression involve disturbances in mood and affect.
   a. This describes schizophrenia.
   b. Genetic research has generated inconclusive evidence, even though genetic factors tend to be stronger for bipolar disorder than for major depression.
   d. Major depression is more common in women; bipolar disorders affect both sexes about equally.
   Knowledge/Psychosocial/Assessment

2. **Correct response: a**
   Research has revealed reduced norepinephrine and serotonin levels in depressive disorder and reduced serotonin and increased norepinephrine levels in bipolar disorder.
   b, c, and d. These altered neurotransmitter levels do not apply to affective disorders.
   Knowledge/Physiologic/Assessment

3. **Correct response: b**
   The cognitive model describes depression as resulting from negative cognition.
   a. The psychoanalytic model attributes depression to the internalization of anger.
   c. The learned helplessness model links loss of control with helplessness.
   d. The integrative model examines the interaction of biochemical, experiential, and behavioral factors.
   Knowledge/Psychosocial/Assessment

4. **Correct response: c**
   To be categorized as a bipolar disorder, there must be at least one manic episode.
   a, b, and d. These describe depressive disorders.
   Knowledge/Psychosocial/Assessment

5. **Correct response: d**
   This patient is viewing her achievement in terms of an "A" being the only passing grade, with any other grade considered a failure (all-or-nothing thinking). She also has established that an "A" is the standard by which she evaluates her achievement (should statements).
   a, b, and c. These negative cognitions do not apply to this situation.
   Application/Psychosocial/Assessment

6. **Correct response: c**
   Internal explanations contribute to reduced self-esteem, stable explanations contribute to the chronic feelings of helplessness, and global explanations contribute to the overall pervasiveness of helplessness.
   a, b, and d. These responses are incorrect because they include either external, unstable, or specific explanations, all of which reduce the likelihood of depression.
   Comprehension/Psychosocial/Assessment

7. **Correct response: b**
   Stable and global explanations and overgeneralizations, a negative cognition, contribute to the process of blowing things out of proportion, to placing too much emphasis on the generality and pervasiveness of negative occurrences.
   a, c, and d. These responses are incorrect in that they contain an unstable explanation, all-or-nothing thinking, or a specific explanation that would contribute to a more circumscribed explanation of the negative occurrence.
   Comprehension/Psychosocial/Assessment

8. **Correct response: d**
   Symptoms of manic behavior include all

those listed under response d as well as those listed under responses a, b, and c—*except* poverty of ideas, apathy, and social isolation, which are typically seen in depressive disorders.

Comprehension/Psychosocial/Assessment

9. **Correct response: b**
   The nurse will need to promote an environment conducive to rest and relaxation (*i.e.,* reducing noise level, dimming light, providing a warm bath, and so forth)
   a. This would represent misuse of restraints.
   c. Providing no intervention would be inappropriate in this case.
   d. This would constitute misuse of isolation.

Application/Safe care/Implementation

10. **Correct response: a**
    The nurse provides alternative behaviors for the unacceptable ones exhibited by the patient for the purpose of assisting the patient to develop self-control. Ideally, the treatment team will have met to discuss alternative behaviors that will be reinforced.
    b. This intervention would be inappropriate because the patient is told only what is unacceptable and is not given any alternatives.
    c. This intervention would be inappropriate because the treatment team's objective is to increase the patient's self-control.
    d. This response in incorrect because the nurse must work in conjunction with the treatment team.

Application/Safe care/Implementation

11. **Correct response: c**
    Hopelessness and previous suicide attempts are the best indicators of suicide.
    a, b, and d. These responses are incorrect because they contain auditory hallucina-

tions, neologisms, and narcissism, respectively. These three are characteristic of psychopathology, and research has shown that suicidal persons usually are not psychotic.

Knowledge/Safe care/Assessment

12. **Correct response: b**
    This approach provides an opportunity for the patient to recognize and label her pain and to begin to develop strategies for effective coping.
    a. This approach does not take into consideration that suicidal persons generally feel hopeless and helpless and are unable to ask for help.
    c and d. These approaches avoid dealing with the issue of suicide, which may communicate the nurse's disinterest and reinforce the patient's feelings of hopelessness. It is a myth that discussing suicide will provoke a suicide attempt.

Application/Safe care/Implementation

13. **Correct response: d**
    The immediate focus is on keeping the patient alive.
    a. This would be an inappropriate plan for a therapeutic relationship.
    b and c. Psychotherapy would assist the patient in achieving the long-term goals listed in these responses.

Application/Psychosocial/Planning

14. **Correct response: a**
    To perform an adequate assessment, the nurse needs thorough and accurate information about the patient's symptoms.
    b, c, and d. Although this information is necessary, none of it would be essential at this point in assessment.

Application/Psychosocial/Assessment

Schizophrenic Disorders

I. Overview

A. Definitions

1. Schizophrenic disorders: a group of related psychotic disorders that involve difficulties in reality testing and relatedness
2. Psychotic disorder: disordered behavior typified by gross impairment of reality testing, personality disintegration, and inability to function

B. Basic concepts

1. Schizophrenia is a severe mental disorder characterized by Bleuler's "four As":
   a. Affect inappropriate to the situation or flat
   b. Associations between thoughts loose or disordered
   c. Autism (withdrawal into one's own self and inner experiences)
   d. Ambivalence or difficulty making choices in decisions, emotions, relationships (e.g., this or that, happy or sad, love or hate)

2. Auditory hallucination (e.g., hearing voices) sometimes is considered the fifth A.
3. Onset of schizophrenia typically occurs in late adolescence to the mid-20s.
4. The course of schizophrenia is variable; onset can be gradual or sudden.
5. The acute phase typically involves psychotic symptoms.
6. Periods of remission often occur, although social and role impairment may persist.
7. About one third of patients recover completely, one third need ongoing prophylactic treatment, and one third have continuing or permanent deterioration.

C. **General characteristics**
1. Common alterations in thought patterns include:
   a. Disjointed, disconnected thinking (loose associations)
   b. Difficulty abstracting
   c. Ideas of reference (believing that things or events in the environment directly relate to self)
2. Perceptual alterations may include:
   a. Heightened or blunted perception
   b. Illusions (misperceptions or exaggeration of environmental stimuli)
   c. Hallucinations (sensory perceptions that are not real—particularly hearing voices)
3. Emotional responses may include:
   a. Restricted expression
   b. Inappropriate affect (not fitting a situation)
   c. Lack of emotional expression (flat affect)
4. Communication problems may involve:
   a. Difficulty communicating clearly (due to problems assimilating and sorting perceptions)
   b. Inappropriate responses to a situation
   c. Irrelevant or wandering responses
   d. Neologisms (made-up words that condense content)
   e. Impoverished responses
5. Possible behavioral alterations include:
   a. Disorganized behavior (aimless or disruptive, not goal-directed)
   b. Peculiarities (ritualistic patterns, unusual movements)
   c. Catatonic posturing (holding bizarre postures for long periods of time)
   d. Catatonic excitement (moving excitedly with no environmental stimuli)

D. **Etiology**
1. The exact cause of schizophrenia remains unclear.

2. Research indicates a potential combination of causative factors: genetic, biochemical, and family or environmental.
3. There is some evidence of genetic transmission; most likely, a vulnerability for the disorder is inherited. Relevant statistics include:
    a. Incidence in the general population: about 1%
    b. Incidence in first-degree relatives (siblings, children) of persons with schizophrenia: 3% to 10%
    c. Incidence in more distant relatives (cousins): about 3%
    d. High incidence (9% to 35%) in both twins if one has schizophrenia, even when they are raised by different parents in different locations
    e. No increased incidence in children adopted into families with a history of schizophrenia
4. Possible evidence of brain alterations and biochemical changes in schizophrenia includes:
    a. Abnormalities in the frontal lobe, which controls motivation and behavioral appropriateness
    b. Enlarged ventricles, which may impair neurologic and social functioning
    c. Poor coordination seen on neurologic tests
    d. Indirect evidence of altered dopamine transmission (the dopamine hypothesis)
    e. Number of biochemical factors still under investigation
5. No evidence clearly indicates that family patterns cause schizophrenia. (Earlier studies had no control groups.)
6. Some evidence suggests that family cohesion and emotional tone can affect the course of the disorder. (This evidence is controversial, however.) Specific factors may include:
    a. Too much cohesion (enmeshment) combined with a negative, critical emotional tone
    b. Negative emotional tone and intrusiveness, associated with higher relapse rates
    c. Unclear or incomplete communication
    d. Family environment inhibiting learning opportunities for coping skills, social controls

E. **Psychosocial implications of schizophrenia**
    1. Psychotic responses indicate impaired reality testing—the patient does not interpret the environment the same way most people do.
    2. Psychotic responses usually are accompanied by lack of insight about the psychotic process—the patient does not perceive the abnormality.
    3. Because of lack of insight, the patient views altered experiences as reality.

4. Patients do not always share their psychotic experiences; the nurse needs to observe for cues.
5. Impairment is manifested in various aspects of the person's functioning (e.g., interpersonal relationships, role functioning, communication).
6. Altered perceptions are frightening to the patient.
7. Altered perceptions can cause the patient to show lack of impulse control.
8. Altered perceptions can cause the patient to withdraw as a way of coping.
9. Changes in the patient's behavior are frightening to the family.
10. Serious mental disorders are stigmatized in society, creating an additional burden for the patient and family.
11. Socioeconomic aspects of a serious mental illness can lead to housing and other related problems.
12. An estimated one third of homeless persons in society have schizophrenia.

II. Types of schizophrenia
A. Disorganized type
1. Characteristics: incoherence, grossly disorganized behavior, flat or very inappropriate affect, grimacing, odd mannerisms, extreme social withdrawal
2. Typically has an early and insidious onset and a chronic course

B. Catatonic type
1. Characteristics: psychomotor disturbances such as catatonic stupor, posturing, or excitement
2. Mutism, malnourishment, exhaustion, self-inflicted injury, or other problems may occur during times of psychomotor disturbance.

C. Paranoid type
1. Characteristics: preoccupation with systematized delusions; auditory hallucinations (e.g., hearing voices)
2. This type is marked by an absence of the disordered behavioral features of disorganized or catatonic types.
3. The patient may exhibit a stilted, formal quality or extreme intensity in interpersonal interactions.
4. Paranoid schizophrenia also involves less social and occupational impairment than do other types.

D. Undifferentiated type
1. Characteristics: a mixture of delusions, hallucinations, incoherence, and disorganized behavior
2. This classification is used when schizophrenia cannot be classified as any of the other types.

    E.   **Residual type**
        1. Characteristics: current absence of acute symptoms but history of past episodes
        2. Typically, the patient exhibits marked social isolation and withdrawal and impaired role functioning.

III. **The nursing process and schizophrenia**
    A.   **Assessment**
        1. Assess the patient's history for precipitating stressors, which may include:
            a. Genetic–biologic vulnerability
            b. Difficult family relationships
            c. Stressful life events
            d. Decreased social competence
            e. Coping skill deficit—overuse of denial and projection
        2. Evaluate for physiologic responses, such as:
            a. Sensory flooding (inability to sort out complex stimuli)
            b. Impaired autonomic response (lack of response to pain or other stimuli)
            c. Altered sleep patterns
            d. Anorexia (may be due to believing food is poisoned)
            e. Abnormal eye blink rate
        3. Assess for typical behavioral responses, including:
            a. Impaired self-care ability
            b. Increased suspiciousness
            c. Impaired communication (e.g., poverty of speech, overelaborate speech, symbolic speech, perseveration, echolalia, neologisms, clang association)
            d. Impaired role functioning
            e. Poor eye contact or overly intense eye contact
            f. Peculiar mannerisms, posturing, echopraxia
            g. Ritualistic behaviors
            h. Immobility and withdrawal
            i. Increased impulsivity
            j. Ambivalence; difficulty in decision making and judgment
        4. Observe for cognitive alterations, particularly:
            a. Poor attention span
            b. Difficulty processing complex stimuli
            c. Preoccupation with internal stimuli or altered perceptions (e.g., having bizarre thoughts, hearing voices)
            d. Magical thinking
            e. Loose associations, flight of ideas
            f. Thought insertion and withdrawal (belief that thoughts can be inserted into or withdrawn from one's head by another)

g.   Confused ego boundaries
h.   Inability to perceive self realistically (lack of insight)
i.   Delusions (paranoid or persecutory, grandiose, somatic, reference)
j.   Hallucinations (auditory, visual, gustatory, tactile)
k.   Illusions (misperceptions of sensory data, social relationships, physical environment)
5.   Also note characteristic affective responses, such as:
a.   Flat or inappropriate affect
b.   Depressed affect
c.   Anger and negativity
d.   Unfocused general anxiety
e.   Emotional ambivalence

B.   Nursing diagnoses
1.   Ineffective Individual Coping:
a.   Related to low self-esteem
b.   Related to inadequate support system
c.   Related to dysfunctional use of defense mechanisms
2.   Social Isolation:
a.   Related to inability to trust
b.   Related to delusional thinking
c.   Related to impaired reality testing
3.   Altered Thought Processes:
a.   Related to impaired ability to process stimuli
b.   Related to genetic and personal vulnerability
c.   Related to severe anxiety

C.   Planning and implementation
1.   For the patient exhibiting withdrawn and seclusive behavior:
a.   Initiate frequent, short, and nondemanding interactions.
b.   Plan simple one-to-one activities and establish a daily routine.
c.   Assume a noncommittal approach to bizarre behavior.
d.   Assist the patient in daily grooming.
e.   Clarify unclear communications (see Display 6–1 for an example).
f.   Introduce patient to group activities gradually.
g.   Assist the patient in goal setting.
h.   Assist the patient with eating if necessary.
i.   Administer neuroleptic medications as prescribed.
2.   For the patient exhibiting paranoid behavior (high suspicion, low trust):
a.   Establish a professional relationship with the patient (being overly friendly may be threatening).
b.   Allow the patient as much control and autonomy as possible.

DISPLAY 6–1.
Clarifying Unclear Communications: An Example

Patient: "The skirts in the sky are flying high and I'm not going with them."

Nurse: "You are trying to tell me something but I don't understand what it is. Can you tell me in a different way?"

Patient: (Points to a nurse walking briskly down the hall) "They're all in a hurry."

Nurse: "You're telling me that the nurses are very busy and that you feel left out?"

Patient: "Yes; I need help with my bath."

Interpretation: In this example, the patient used highly symbolic language in trying to communicate. The nurse indicates that she does not understand what is being said. When the patient tries again, the nurse thinks she understands and checks out what she hears with the patient. The patient then confirms the message.

---

    c.   Establish trust through short interactions that communicate your interest and concern.

    d.   Explain treatments, medications, laboratory tests, and other procedures in a clear, direct manner.

    e.   Encourage the patient's involvement in ongoing support systems (e.g., work, family, friends, community).

    f.   Do not focus on or reinforce the patient's suspicious thoughts and delusions.

    g.   Identify and respond to the patient's emotional needs underlying suspicious thoughts or delusions (see Display 6–2 for an example).

    h.   Handle the patient's refusal of medications by taking a firm, matter-of-fact approach.

  3.   For the patient experiencing hallucinations or delusions:

    a.   Do not reinforce hallucinations or delusions by discussing or agreeing with them while they are occurring.

DISPLAY 6–2.
Responding to Suspicious Thoughts or Delusions: An Example

Patient: (Standing by the Nurses' Station, looking at the tape recorder on the desk) "That tape recorder you have is used to record my thoughts. People here are against me." (Appears furtive and suspicious)

Nurse: "It doesn't seem to me that this is so. This tape recorder is used to record the night nurse's report. I believe that you're safe here."

Patient: I don't feel safe here. Can I stay by the desk while you are here?"

Nurse: "Yes; I'll be here for 5 more minutes until lunch trays come. Here's a newspaper for you to read."

Patient: (Remains by the Nurses' Station and reads the paper)

Interpretation: In this example, the patient misinterprets the environment by drawing an unwarranted conclusion about the tape recorder kept at the Nurses' Station. The nurse responds by presenting reality to the patient in a matter-of-fact manner. She also responds to the underlying meaning of the patient's communication by saying that the patient is safe here and by allowing him to remain close to her. She refocuses the patient on another environmental object, the newspaper.

b. Point out that you do not share the patient's perception (e.g., "I don't hear the voices you say you hear").

c. Do not argue with the patient about the hallucinations or delusions.

d. Respond to the feelings or message the patient is conveying (e.g., "You seem frightened").

e. Redirect and focus the patient on a structured activity.

f. Move the patient to a quieter, less stimulating environment.

g. Wait until the patient is not experiencing hallucinations or delusions before providing patient teaching about them.

h. Explain that hallucinations or delusions are symptoms of psychiatric disorders.

i. Point out that factors within the patient (e.g., anxiety) or within the environment (e.g., excessive stimuli) may stimulate hallucinations.

j. Help the patient control hallucinations by refocusing on reality and taking prescribed neuroleptic medications.

k. Help the patient learn to "live with" hallucinations (such as hearing voices) by giving them less status in his or her life.

4. For the patient exhibiting agitated behavior and potential for violence:

a. Always work with other staff to manage agitated, impulsive patients.

b. Assess the patient's potential for violence; observe for cues of escalation when agitated behavior begins.

c. Provide a safe, quiet environment; decrease stimuli.

d. Provide a safe outlet for energy and anger (e.g., letting the patient shout, pace, or throw soft objects).

e. Discourage competitive activities.

f. Set limits on unacceptable behavior.

g. Do not retaliate if the patient is verbally hostile.

h. Isolate the patient from the general milieu if agitation increases.

i. Administer p.r.n. medications when necessary.

j. If restraints are necessary, apply them in a safe and nonpunitive manner.

k. For a patient in restraints, follow protocols and provide safe care.

D. Evaluation

1. The patient states awareness of precipitating stressors and ways to reduce or minimize them.

2. Physiologic outcomes

a. The patient demonstrates increased ability to handle complex stimuli.

    b.   The patient exhibits response to autonomic threats (e.g., pain).

    c.   The patient exhibits improved sleep patterns.

    d.   The patient demonstrates increased food intake.

    e.   The patient demonstrates appropriate eye contact during conversations.

3.   Behavioral outcomes

    a.   The patient demonstrates improved self-care abilities.

    b.   The patient exhibits decreased paranoid behaviors or beliefs.

    c.   The patient exhibits improved communication patterns.

    d.   The patient displays age- and preparation-appropriate role functions.

    e.   The patient exhibits reduced peculiar mannerisms.

    f.   The patient demonstrates decreased ritualistic behavior patterns.

    g.   The patient exhibits decreased immobility and withdrawal.

    h.   The patient exhibits increased physical and social activity.

    i.   The patient demonstrates improved impulse control.

4.   Cognitive outcomes

    a.   The patient exhibits increased attention span.

    b.   The patient demonstrates improved ability to process complex stimuli.

    c.   The patient begins to focus on external events rather than on internal concerns.

    d.   The patient exhibits decreased or controlled magical thinking, delusions, hallucinations, and illusions.

    e.   The patient displays more connected and appropriate thought patterns.

    f.   The patient reports increased self-awareness.

5.   Affective outcomes

    a.   The patient displays more appropriate affect in relation to own feelings and social contacts.

    b.   The patient exhibits reduced anger and negativity.

    c.   The patient expresses emotions appropriately.

Bibliography

American Psychiatric Association (1987). *Diagnostic and statistical manual of mental disorders (DSM-III-R)* (3rd ed., revised). Washington, DC: Author.

Doenges, M., Townsend, M., & Moorehouse, M. (1988). *Psychiatric care plans: Guidelines for client care.* Philadelphia: F. A. Davis.

Gerace, L. (1988). Schizophrenia and the family: Nursing implications. *Archives of Psychiatric Nursing,* II*(3),* 141–145.

Johnson, B. S. (1989). *Psychiatric-mental health nursing: Adaptation and growth* (2nd ed.). Philadelphia: J. B. Lippincott.

Stuart, G. W., & Sundeen, S. J. (1987). *Principles and practice of psychiatric nursing* (3rd ed.). St. Louis: C. V. Mosby.

Torrey, E. F. (1983). *Surviving schizophrenia: A family manual.* New York: Harper & Row.

Wilson, H. S., & Kneisl, C. R. (1988). *Psychiatric nursing* (3rd ed.). Menlo Park, CA: Addison-Wesley.

STUDY QUESTIONS

1. Which type of schizophrenia is characterized by deteriorated behavior and extreme social withdrawal?
   a. disorganized
   b. catatonic
   c. paranoid
   d. undifferentiated

2. Which of the following statements regarding genetic transmission of schizophrenia is true?
   a. No evidence exists suggesting genetic transmission of schizophrenia.
   b. The incidence of schizophrenia is the same in all families, regardless of family history of schizophrenia.
   c. Twin and adoption studies indicate that the vulnerability for schizophrenia may be inherited.
   d. Conclusive evidence indicates that a specific gene transmits schizophrenia.

3. Mr. Adams has been newly diagnosed with paranoid schizophrenia. When planning care, which expected changes in Mr. Adams' perceptions should the nurse keep in mind?
   a. He will believe that he is not functioning normally and will constantly ask for help.
   b. He often will misinterpret environmental stimuli.
   c. He will notice no changes in either himself or the environment.
   d. He will act in a socially appropriate manner.

4. Which of the following nursing actions would be indicated for Mr. Adams?
   a. spending a great deal of time with him
   b. establishing a nondemanding relationship with him
   c. encouraging him to become involved in group rather than individual activities
   d. leaving him alone until he initiates a relationship

5. Mr. Adams believes that his medicines are dangerous and says he does not want to take them. Which of the following actions should the nurse take first?
   a. Hand him the medications and firmly instruct him to take them.
   b. Ask why he thinks the medicines are dangerous.
   c. Ask if he would rather have an injection.
   d. Withhold the medications until he is less suspicious.

6. Ms. Gullickson, a 20-year-old single woman, is admitted to the psychiatric unit because, as her mother states, she "has been behaving more and more strangely"—secluding herself in her bedroom, no longer showering or dressing, eating with her hands instead of utensils, and responding to others' attempts at communication with only mumbling and inappropriate grinning.

   Her mother reports that Ms. Gullickson always has been "sensitive and immature" and "a loner." Based on these assessment data, which nursing diagnosis would be of primary importance for this patient?
   a. High Risk for Violence: Self-Directed
   b. Dysfunctional Grieving
   c. Anxiety
   d. Social Isolation

7. Which of the following statements regarding age of onset of schizophrenia in Ms. Gullickson is correct?
   a. Age of onset is typical for schizophrenia.
   b. Age of onset is later than usual for schizophrenia.
   c. Age of onset is earlier than usual for schizophrenia.
   d. Age of onset follows no predictable pattern in schizophrenia.

8. When planning Ms. Gullickson's care, the nurse should recognize that withdrawn behavior provides a way for Ms. Gullickson to

a. avoid developing mature relationships

b. cope with altered thoughts and perceptions

c. remain preoccupied with bizarre delusions

d. prevent her family from interfering

9. An appropriate nursing strategy to deal with Ms. Gullickson's withdrawal would be

a. Do not attempt to establish a relationship.

b. Make group interactions the main focus of therapy.

c. Hold in-depth one-to-one counseling sessions.

d. Keep interactions short, frequent, and nondemanding.

10. When evaluating Ms. Gullickson's care, the nurse should keep in mind which of the following points?

a. Frequent reassessment is needed based on her response to treatment.

b. The family need not be included in the care because she is not a minor.

c. She is too ill to learn about her illness.

d. Relapse is not an issue for a patient like her.

11. Mr. Kenson, a 27-year-old man with paranoid schizophrenia, has been on the unit for several days. He remains aloof and suspicious, and his grooming and self-care are excellent. His family reports that he lives at home and holds a clerical job in the nearby hospital. Mr. Kenson periodically looks intently toward the ceiling and cocks his head to one side while tugging at his ear. In assessing this behavior, the nurse should consider that Mr. Kenson

a. has peculiar mannerisms

b. may be hearing voices

c. is avoiding the nurse

d. is daydreaming

12. One afternoon, Mr. Kenson becomes upset, reporting that an item of clothing is missing from his room. Which of the following actions should the nurse take first?

a. Tell Mr. Kenson that theft is common in hospitals.

b. Report to the staff that the item is missing.

c. Suggest that Mr. Kenson be more careful with his clothing.

d. Ask Mr. Kenson where he has looked for the item.

13. While talking with the nurse, Mr. Kenson states that the FBI is monitoring and recording his every movement and that microphones have been implanted in the unit walls for this purpose. Which of the following nursing actions would be most therapeutic in response to this revelation?

a. Confront the delusional material directly by telling Mr. Kenson that this simply is not so.

b. Tell Mr. Kenson that this must seem frightening to him but that you believe he is safe here.

c. Tell Mr. Kenson to wait and talk about these beliefs in his one-to-one counseling sessions.

d. Isolate Mr. Kenson when he begins to talk about these beliefs.

14. Which of the following behaviors recorded in Mr. Kenson's chart could indicate a potential for violence?

a. increased agitation and hostility; hallucinations

b. withdrawal to room; quiet and brooding manner

c. talking about discharge; calling family members often

d. assisting with unit clean-up; talking to other patients

15. After treatment, Mr. Kenson's condition improves; he is now ready to return to his job as an assistant in the medical records department of his neighborhood hospital. During discharge planning, the staff evaluates several placement possibilities for Mr. Kenson. Which of the following placements most likely would be beneficial?

a. home with his family where he shares a bedroom with his teenage brother

b. a rented room on the same street where his family lives

c. a large halfway house in the center of the city in which his family lives
d. a state institution about an hour's drive away from where his family lives

ANSWER KEY

1. **Correct response: a**
   Disorganized schizophrenia is the more insidious type of schizophrenia. The patient becomes regressed and disorganized in his total behavior, thinking, and communication.
   b, c, and d. These types of schizophrenia have different characteristics.
   Knowledge/Psychosocial/Assessment

2. **Correct response: c**
   Research indicates that a variety of factors apparently contributes to schizophrenia, one of these being genetic vulnerability.
   a. Studies show a genetic pattern to the disease.
   b. The incidence of schizophrenia is higher in persons whose immediate family has a history of schizophrenia.
   d. Such specific evidence has not yet been found.
   Knowledge/Physiologic/Analysis (Dx)

3. **Correct response: b**
   Patients with paranoid symptoms believe that something is wrong or dangerous in others or in the environment and act accordingly.
   a. In most psychotic illnesses, self-insight into changes is lacking.
   c. The patient does notice that things are changing, and as a result, his behavior also changes.
   d. Socially inappropriate behavior commonly results from misinterpretation of the environment.
   Application/Psychosocial/Planning

4. **Correct response: b**
   Too much friendliness, intensity, and warmth may be threatening to a paranoid patient. It is best to keep interactions short and to maintain a professional distance.
   a. This approach would be too intense.
   c. A paranoid patient does better in individual activities until a sense of trust has developed.
   d. This would cause the nurse to avoid the patient, an undesirable approach.
   Application/Safe care/Implementation

5. **Correct response: a**
   It is best to take a matter-of-fact, firm attitude when trying to get a paranoid patient to take his medications. If the nurse appears uncertain, this will add to the patient's insecurity and fear.
   b. The nurse already knows that Mr. Adams believes his medicines are dangerous; this response would only reinforce his beliefs.
   c. This action may make him feel more threatened.
   d. Withholding medications prescribed to relieve paranoia will cause exacerbation of paranoid thoughts and feelings.
   Application/Safe care/Implementation

6. **Correct response: d**
   Ms. Gullickson manifests social withdrawal, which is related to the general behavioral deterioration and inappropriate affect typical of disorganized schizophrenia.
   a, b, and c. These nursing diagnoses are more often associated with other psychiatric conditions and are not implied in the data given about Ms. Gullickson.
   Comprehension/Psychosocial/Analysis (Dx)

7. **Correct response: a**
   The primary age of onset for schizophrenia is late adolescence through young adulthood (age 17 to 27). Paranoid schizophrenia may sometimes have a later onset.
   b, c, and d. These responses are all incorrect.
   Knowledge/Health promotion/Assessment

8. **Correct response: b**

Withdrawal represents a way for the patient to defend against the confusion engendered by overwhelming sensory stimuli that she cannot process normally.

   a and c. These are secondary effects of withdrawal.

   d. The scenario does not present sufficient information to warrant this conclusion.

Comprehension/Psychosocial/Planning

9. *Correct response: d*

The nurse must proceed slowly and build trust gradually with a patient like Ms. Gullickson, initiating contact by showing interest in her daily activities, hygiene, and so forth.

   a. This approach suggests ignoring the patient, which would be inappropriate.

   b and c. These approaches likely would be overwhelming to Ms. Gullickson.

Application/Safe care/Implementation

10. *Correct response: a*

Because patients respond to treatment in different ways, the nurse must constantly evaluate the patient and her potentials. Premorbid adjustment is another fact to consider.

   b. Most patients with schizophrenia go home, and the family should be involved and supported.

   c. Ms. Gullickson can learn certain things about her illness if information is given gradually and in terms that she can understand.

   d. Relapses are common in schizophrenia.

Application/Psychosocial/Evaluation

11. *Correct response: b*

Patients with paranoid schizophrenia often hear voices; this behavior would indicate that this might be true for Mr. Kenson.

   a. A mannerism is usually an involuntary repetitive movement.

   c and d. These are less specific responses.

Application/Psychosocial/Assessment

12. *Correct response: d*

By staying calm and asking Mr. Kenson this question, the nurse is communicating the ordinary nature of this type of event. A suspicious patient often jumps to unwarranted conclusions; perhaps he has not looked carefully for the item before reporting it missing.

   a. This response would tend to add to any unsafe feelings the patient has.

   b. This should not be done until after looking for the item.

   c. This is a moralistic, materialistic response.

Analysis/Psychosocial/Implementation

13. *Correct response: b*

The nurse must realize that these perceptions are very real to the patient. Acknowledging the patient's feelings provides support; explaining that she herself doesn't see the situation in the same way provides reality orientation.

   a. The direct approach will not work with this patient and may decrease trust.

   c. This approach will reinforce the delusion.

   d. Isolation will increase anxiety. Distraction with a radio or activities would be a better approach.

Application/Psychosocial/Implementation

14. *Correct response: a*

Indicators of a possible violent episode include increased motor activity, frightening or threatening delusions or hallucinations, verbal hostility.

   b. These are not generally indicators of escalating violence.

   c and d. These behaviors are associated with clinical improvement.

Application/Safe care/Assessment

15. *Correct response: b*

Because Mr. Kenson has a tendency toward aloofness and suspicion, yet is fairly functional, the best placement would be independent but near his family so he can get support.

a. Mr. Kenson is not flexible enough to live with a teenager.

c. Living in a large facility would not be as productive for a patient like Mr. Kenson.

d. Mr. Kenson has too many strengths to be institutionalized.

Analysis/Psychosocial/Evaluation

Alterations in Human Sexuality

7

I. Overview

A. Definitions

1. Concepts related to human sexuality include:
   a. A sense of maleness or femaleness (gender identity)
   b. Desire for contact, warmth, tenderness, love
   c. Encompassing the total sense of self
   d. Integral part of life
   e. Evident in a person's manner of relating

    2.   Aspects of sexual health include:
- a. Integration of somatic, intellectual, and social aspects of sexual being
- b. Constantly changing and evolving
- c. Falling within a wide range of expression
- d. Determined by the individual
- e. Determined by local community and society at large

    3.   Gender identity involves:
- a. Personal or private sense of identity as masculine, feminine, or ambivalent
- b. Sex role assignment

B.   **Theories of sexuality**

    1.   Historical perspective
- a. Past sexual behavior patterns influence present concepts of sexuality.
- b. Certain Christian doctrines of sex outside of marriage and for purposes other than procreation as sinful exert a pervasive influence on contemporary societal attitudes.
- c. Myths and misconceptions such as "women are pure" and "nice girls don't do that" also influence societal attitudes.
- d. The women's rights movement has challenged traditional views of women as passive sexual beings.
- e. Masters and Johnson's work has helped promote a new freedom of sexual expression.
- f. Kinsey and colleagues' work has proposed a continuum of human sexuality and sexual expression.
- g. The sexual revolution linked improved contraception methods and changing societal attitudes with increased openness of sexual expression.

    2.   Psychoanalytic perspective
- a. Freud suggested that an interplay of heredity, biology, and social factors influence a person's sexuality.
- b. Sexuality is important to personality development.
- c. Children are sexual beings; Oedipus and Electra conflicts explain the developmental issue of sexual attraction to the opposite-sex parent.

    3.   Behavioral perspective
- a. Sexual behavior is learned and reinforced from life experiences.
- b. Examination of sexual behavior aids understanding of sociocultural, ethnic, and gender issues.
- c. Treatment for sexual disorders is based on direct intervention.

    4.   Social perspective
- a. Modes of sexual expression are learned.

      b.   Sexual expression is influenced by gender identity and gender roles.

      c.   The acceptability of sexual behaviors is influenced by societal values.

  5.   Actuarial perspective

      a.   Information about sexual behavior and attitudes is gathered from demographic data, surveys, and interviews.

      b.   Obtaining statistically complete and accurate data is often difficult.

  6.   Sociologic perspective

      a.   Sexual behavior is influenced by social conditioning.

      b.   Social movements—such as the women's rights and gay rights movements—influence societal attitudes regarding sexuality and sexual expression.

  7.   Cultural perspective

      a.   Widely divergent patterns of sexuality are seen in various world cultures.

      b.   Tolerance of individual differences can be enhanced through cross-cultural understanding.

  8.   Biologic perspective

      a.   Various biochemical, hormonal, vascular, neuromuscular, and anatomic factors influence sexuality and sexual expression.

      b.   Sexual response involves a combination of biologic, psychosocial, and cultural variables.

  9.   Developmental perspective

      a.   Childhood involves issues of gender identity and developing sexuality.

      b.   Adolescence presents concerns about sexual development and intimacy.

      c.   Reproduction issues (e.g., fertility–infertility, contraception, childbirth) commonly become important during young and middle adulthood.

      d.   The aging process raises issues related to response and expression.

C. **Sexual anatomy**

  1.   Female genitalia include:

      a.   Clitoris: highly sensitive to touch; primary function is to receive and transmit sexual stimuli

      b.   Mons and labia: sensitive to pressure and touch

      c.   Vagina: sensitive to stretch; outer third is the most sensitive area.

  2.   Male genitalia include:

      a.   Penis: glans highly sensitive to touch; shaft also sensitive to touch

      b.   Scrotum: skin sensitive to touch

        3.   Other sexual organs and structures include the lips, tongue, anus, buttocks, breasts, and skin in general.

  D. **Sexual response cycle**

      1.   Desire phase

          a.   Libido

          b.   Receptivity to sexual activity or interaction

          c.   Triggered by physical, psychologic, and environmental factors

      2.   Excitement phase

          a.   Female lubrication

          b.   Male and female vasocongestion

          c.   Male erection

      3.   Plateau

          a.   High state of sexual arousal before orgasm

          b.   Orgasmic platform with narrowing of vaginal opening

          c.   Clitoris engorged and retracted

          d.   Head of penis (glans) somewhat larger

          e.   Clear fluid emitted from penis

      4.   Orgasm phase

          a.   Reflex triggered by a high state of sexual arousal

          b.   Rhythmic contractions of pelvic organs and muscles

          c.   Controlled by spinal nerve centers

          d.   In women, clitoral or vaginal stimulation possibly preceding orgasm

          e.   For men, two stages of orgasm: emission of semen into urethra and ejaculation of semen out of urethra

      5.   Resolution phase

          a.   Organs back to normal

          b.   Male refractory period: cannot reach orgasm again without waiting

          c.   Female: no refractory period, allowing for multiple orgasms

          d.   Phase possibly 30 minutes long

  E. **Dimensions of sexuality**

      1.   Healthy dimension of sexuality: normal sexual behavior

          a.   Consensual and mutually satisfying

          b.   Between two consenting adults

          c.   Not forceful

          d.   Private

          e.   Not psychologically or physically harmful

          f.   Example: mutually pleasurable heterosexual or homosexual behavior

      2.   Mild alteration in the dimension of sexuality: sexual behavior impaired by anxiety stemming from:

          a.   Personal judgment

        b.   Societal judgment
3. Moderate alteration in the dimension of sexuality: dysfunction in sexual performance
        a.   Sexual arousal disorders
        b.   Orgasmic disorders
        c.   Sexual desire disorders
4. Moderate to severe alteration in the dimension of sexuality: gender dysfunctions
        a.   Transsexualism
        b.   Gender identity disorder of childhood
5. Severe alteration in the dimension of sexuality: harmful, forceful, or nonprivate sex
        a.   Pedophilia
        b.   Exhibitionism
        c.   Sexual sadism

F. Factors associated with gender development
1. Biologic imperative: gender based on anatomy
2. Cognitive switch: cognitive labeling of own sex at age 3 or 4
3. Social learning and labeling
        a.   Gender identity continuously constructed and maintained through lifetime
        b.   Stability dependent on social expectations, demands, and feedback regarding self

G. Characteristic patterns of sexual expression or orientation
1. Heterosexuality considered the norm (in the United States) in the past (more recently, norm may also encompass homosexual and bisexual behavior)
        a.   Erotic attraction to opposite sex
        b.   A sexual majority
        c.   Sexual behaviors especially include penetration of penis into vagina
2. Heterosexual–homosexual continuum: the Kinsey scale
        a.   A seven-point scale (0–6)
        b.   Exclusively heterosexual experience rated 0
        c.   Exclusively homosexual behavior rated 6
        d.   Bisexual between 1 and 5 or 2 and 4
        e.   Ratings based on behavior and fantasies
3. Homosexuality
        a.   Erotic attraction to same sex
        b.   A sexual minority
        c.   Estimate 10% of U.S. population
        d.   No cause established
        e.   Psychologic, emotional, sexual functioning normal
        f.   Includes those with homosexual fantasies
        g.   An emotional preference

       h.   A social role
       i.   Part of one's identity
       j.   Gay and lesbian subculture a major social support
       k.   Necessary to "come out" to join subculture
       l.   Varied cultural, social, and sexual aspects
       m.   Some use of exaggerated mannerisms and dress

4. Male homosexuality
    a.   Sexual behaviors especially include fellatio, anal intercourse, manual stimulation
    b.   AIDS epidemic concerns
    c.   Currently using lower-risk behaviors

5. Lesbianism
    a.   Sexual behaviors especially include cunnilingus, mutual masturbation, rubbing genitals against other's body
    b.   Some lesbians assume "butch" and "femme" roles
    c.   Some use neither feminine nor masculine role
    d.   Lesbian communities: bars, overt feminist activist groups, communes, and so forth

6. Bisexuality
    a.   Sexual attraction to members of both sexes
    b.   Percent of population not documented
    c.   Not well studied

II. Types of sexual alterations
A. Alterations in gender identity
1. Transsexualism
    a.   Persistent discomfort about one's sex assignment
    b.   Feeling of being trapped in the wrong body
    c.   Persistent preoccupation with eliminating one's primary and secondary sex characteristics
    d.   Two or more years' duration
    e.   Caused by confused learning about gender roles
    f.   Influenced by fetal sex hormones
    g.   Sex-change surgery often sought
    h.   Functioning reportedly improved in two thirds of patients after surgery

2. Gender identity disorder of childhood
    a.   Persistent and intense distress at one's sex
    b.   Person insists that he or she is the opposite sex
    c.   Preoccupation with other sex's clothing and behavior
    d.   Assertion that he or she will grow up to have sexual anatomy of the other sex
    e.   Girls: reject sitting for urination
    f.   Boys: say testes will disappear
    g.   Cross-dressing may precede the disorder

3. Nontranssexual cross-gender disorder
    a.   Persistent discomfort about one's sex

        b.   No preoccupation with ridding self of genitals

B.   **Alterations in sexual orientation**
    1.   Ego-dystonic homosexuality involves:
        a.   Weak heterosexual arousal with desired heterosexual relationships
        b.   An unwanted homosexual arousal pattern
        c.   A DSM-III-R diagnosis
        d.   Past medical opinion: all homosexuality an illness
        e.   Current diagnosis dependent on an unwanted pattern (ego-dystonic)
    2.   Some psychiatric thinking continues classification of homosexuality as an illness, which is inconsistent with DSM-III-R criteria

C.   **Alterations in sexual behavior**
    1.   Sexual acting-out
        a.   Sexual behavior disturbance
        b.   Disturbed conduct or impulse control
        c.   Making sexually provocative remarks
        d.   Inappropriate flirting
        e.   Inappropriate sexual touching of others
        f.   Public masturbation
        g.   Public exhibition of genitals
        h.   Extramarital affairs
        i.   Promiscuity
        j.   Testing of sexual attractiveness
        k.   Presence of inadequate coping and interpersonal skills
        l.   An attempt to alleviate intense anxiety
        m.   High sexual drive
        n.   Guilt: may or may not be present
    2.   Paraphilia
        a.   A specific object or activity required for full sexual arousal and satisfaction
        b.   Usually male
        c.   Behavior often followed by guilt, shame, low self-esteem, or anxiety
        d.   Causes not clearly known
        e.   Exhibitionism: intense sexual arousal or desire derived from exhibiting genitals
        f.   Voyeurism: intense sexual arousal or desire when observing nakedness or sexual activity
        g.   Sexual sadism: intense sexual arousal or desire when inflicting suffering
        h.   Sexual masochism: intense sexual arousal or desire when made to suffer
        i.   Fetishism: intense sexual arousal or desire associated with inanimate articles (e.g., clothing)

        j.   Transvestic fetishism: intense sexual arousal or desire of male when dressed in female clothing
        k.   Zoophilia: intense sexual arousal or desire with animals
        l.   Frotteurism: intense sexual arousal or desire when rubbing against a nonconsenting person
        m.   Other paraphilias (e.g., necrophilia: corpse; telephone scatologia: lewdness)

  3. Pedophilia
        a.   Adult sexual arousal with children
        b.   Nonconsensual sex
        c.   Usually committed by a familiar person, such as a family member or friend
        d.   A paraphilia
        e.   A crime

  4. Victims of pedophilia
        a.   Disturbed sleeping, eating, playing
        b.   Regressive behavior
        c.   Angry outbursts
        d.   Withdrawal

D. Alterations in sexual functioning: general
  1. Sexual dysfunction
        a.   Unsatisfying changes in sexual function
        b.   Both physical and psychologic origins
        c.   Organic causes: drugs, neuromuscular diseases, endocrine disorders, etc.
        d.   Emotional influences: anxiety, guilt, fear
        e.   Cause: may be relationship conflicts and communication
        f.   Generalized dysfunction: in all sexual situations
        g.   Situational dysfunction: in selected situations or activities

  2. Disorders of sexual desire
        a.   Hypoactive sexual desire: absence of sexual fantasies and desires
        b.   Sexual aversion disorder: avoidance of genital sexual contact with a partner

  3. Sexual arousal disorder
        a.   Failure to attain and maintain erection
        b.   Lack of lubrication (female)
        c.   Persistent or recurrent lack of subjective sense of sexual excitement and pleasure
        d.   Physical or psychologic origin
        e.   One third of erectile problems caused by organic problems
        f.   Most caused by fear and anxiety about sexual performance
        g.   Spectator role: noninvolved, evaluative attitude during sexual activity
        h.   Reduced spontaneity with objective intellectual thinking

    i.   Without emotional and physical arousal, no erection and lubrication
    j.   Relationship causes (e.g., inadequate communication about sexual needs)
4. Orgasm disorders: inhibited male and female orgasm
    a.   Absence or delay of orgasm after normal sexual arousal phase
    b.   Sexual stimulation adequate in intensity and duration
5. Female orgasm disorders: inhibited orgasm
    a.   Preorgasmic women: special category for those having not yet learned to have orgasm
    b.   Common problem for women to have orgasmic concerns
    c.   Diagnosis requires that adequate sexual stimulation be present
    d.   Normal variation for women to have orgasm during sexual play but not during intercourse
    e.   Physical causes: hormonal, illness, drugs
    f.   Psychologic causes: lack of information, negative attitudes, anxiety, fear, guilt, fear of pregnancy
    g.   Other psychologic causes: fear of loss of control, excessive vulnerability
    h.   Sociocultural causes: women who believe their sexual role is passive
6. Male orgasm disorders: premature ejaculation
    a.   Ejaculation before, upon, or shortly after penetration
    b.   Ejaculation occurs before patient or partner wants
    c.   Dependent on partner and patient definition
    d.   Causes not substantiated empirically
    e.   Early conditioning of rapid ejaculation a possible cause
    f.   Inability to perceive arousal level accurately
    g.   Lowered sensory threshold from infrequent sex
7. Male orgasm disorders: inhibited orgasm
    a.   Infrequent incidence
    b.   Erection maintained for a long period (e.g., 1 hour)
    c.   Persistent or recurrent delay in or absence of ejaculation
    d.   Neuromuscular diseases (e.g., multiple sclerosis) a cause
    e.   Anxiety and guilt possible psychologic causes
    f.   Fear of pregnancy, performance pressure other possible psychologic causes
E. **Alterations in sexual functioning: painful disorders**
    1. Vaginismus
        a.   An involuntary vaginal spasm at penetration
        b.   Penetration painful or impossible
        c.   Spasm present on pelvic exam
        d.   Partner fears hurting her
        e.   Sexual disorder may develop in partner as a reaction

      f.   Causes: protection against anticipated pain
      g.   Associated with sexual trauma, intense guilt, high religiosity

  2. Dyspareunia
      a.   Painful intercourse
      b.   Often due to physical causes
      c.   Vaginal and glans penis infections and irritations a cause
      d.   Medications that dry lubrication a cause
      e.   Pelvic disorders a cause
      f.   Results in negative emotions
      g.   Anticipation of pain decreases pleasure

F. Alterations in sexual functioning due to drugs and surgery

  1. Medications that can impair sexual function include:
      a.   Antianxiety agents: changes in sexual desire
      b.   Anti-parkinsonism drugs: desire and ejaculatory changes
      c.   Antipsychotic agents: desire, erection, lubrication, orgasm, breast, menstrual changes
      d.   Tricyclic antidepressants: breast, testicular, desire, erection, lubrication, orgasm changes
      e.   Monoamine oxidase inhibitors: desire, erection, lubrication, orgasm changes
      f.   Antihypertensives: arousal and orgasm inhibition
      g.   Steroid therapy: desire increase
      h.   Antihistamines: lubrication inhibition
      i.   Testosterone: desire increase
      j.   Estrogen: female lubrication increase, male arousal and orgasm inhibition
      k.   Antabuse: orgasm delay

  2. Effects of alcohol abuse and nontherapeutic drugs on sexuality include:
      a.   Alcohol, barbiturates, and narcotics (heroin, morphine, codeine, and methadone): depress the CNS, which decreases libido and sexual responses
      b.   Stimulants (amphetamines and cocaine): enhance libido when used in acute doses
      c.   Amphetamines: diminish libido and sexual functioning when used in chronic doses
      d.   Hallucinogens (LSD, DMT, mescaline, THC): have variable effects on sexuality, including enhancement, no effect, and impaired sexual functioning
      e.   Cantharides (Spanish fly): may cause priapism by irritating the genitourinary tract
      f.   Amyl nitrate: promotes genital vascular responses and is reported to improve orgasms

  3. Surgeries that can affect sexuality include:
      a.   Organ loss (e.g., hysterectomy)

      b.   Body part loss (e.g., penectomy)
      c.   Body function loss (e.g., nerve transmission)
      d.   Body orifice change (e.g., colostomy)

G.   **Alterations in sexual functioning due to the aging process**
    1.   Female menopause involves such changes as vaginal atrophy and decreased lubrication.
    2.   Changes in elderly men include:
      a.   Decreased testosterone levels
      b.   The need for more direct genital stimulation
      c.   Decreased erectile firmness
      d.   Less intense orgasm
      e.   Increased refractory time
    3.   Elderly persons of either sex often experience decreased sexual activity due to such factors as sexual boredom, disinterest, impaired physical condition, cultural inhibition, and physical attrition from disuse.

H.   **Sexual addictions**
    1.   Recurrent, compulsive, self-destructive behavior
    2.   Includes promiscuity, compulsive masturbation, voyeurism, exhibitionism, pedophilia
    3.   Pattern includes preoccupation, ritualization, compulsive sexual behaviors, and despair
    4.   Development of addiction
      a.   First, acting out inner conflict or stress
      b.   Second, acting on the addiction for its own sake

III. **Nursing process in sexual alterations**
  A.   Assessment
    1.   Sexual history should include information on:
      a.   Past learning about sex
      b.   Past sexual experiences
      c.   Health or illness status and sexual function
      d.   Medication effects
      e.   Birth control concerns
      f.   Discomfort during sex
      g.   Concerns about masturbation, homosexuality, and so forth
    2.   Important physiologic data include:
      a.   Physiologic data, laboratory data, medications
      b.   Nocturnal penile tumescence
      c.   Vaginal plethysmography
      d.   Physical examination findings
    3.   Dimensions of sexuality to consider include:
      a.   Gender identity
      b.   Sexual orientation
      c.   Sexual behavior

           d.   Sexual functioning

           e.   Phases of sexual response cycle

  4.   Summary of sex problems or concerns should include:

           a.   Patient's description

           b.   When problem started

           c.   Frequency of occurrence

           d.   Circumstances at occurrence

           e.   Patient's ideas about cause

           f.   Effect on partner

           g.   Patient's efforts at solving problem

  5.   Evaluation of precipitating stressors should explore:

           a.   Stress or change: new job, relocation, new child

           b.   Emotional or physical illness

           c.   Hospitalization, surgery

           d.   Body changes (disfiguration, hormonal)

           e.   Pain

           f.   Medication use

  6.   Assessment of coping measures should cover:

           a.   Fantasy

           b.   Projection: blaming partner for difficulties

           c.   Denial of sexual problems

           d.   Rationalization

           e.   Withdrawal from sexual activity

B. **Analysis and nursing diagnoses**

  1.   The nurse dealing with sexuality issues needs knowledge of sexual function–dysfunction and the range of sexual practices.

  2.   The nurse also must develop self-awareness concerning personal values, biases, and comfort level with sexuality.

  3.   Another important factor is awareness of the interrelationship between physiologic, emotional, and sociocultural variables in sexuality.

  4.   Pertinent North American Nursing Diagnosis Association (NANDA) diagnoses may include:

           a.   Altered Sexuality Patterns

           b.   Sexual Dysfunction

           c.   Disturbance in Self-Concept: Body Image, Self-Esteem, Personal Identity

           d.   Altered Family Processes

           e.   Ineffective Coping

C. **Planning and implementation**

  1.   Levels of nurse intervention include:

           a.   Life experience sharing: minimally professional and effective

           b.   Basic intervention, involving:

                (1)   Basic knowledge of sexual function

          (2)   Self-awareness
          (3)   Nonjudgmental attitude
          (4)   Effective facilitation of patient sharing and problem solving (use of nursing process)

    c.   Intermediate level, involving:
          (1)   Synthesis of knowledge, self-awareness, communication skills, and problem solving (use of nursing process)
          (2)   Validation of varying sexual norms and practices
          (3)   Teaching about sexual functioning, with some specific direction, suggestion, or problem-solving with patient (counseling)

    d.   Advanced level (sex therapy especially focused on serious sexual problems and gender disorders), encompassing:
          (1)   Standards determined by American Association of Sex Educators, Counselors, and Therapists (AASECT)
          (2)   Permission or acceptance of sexual behavior (as long as not harmful or illegal)
          (3)   Information and education about sexual functioning
          (4)   Facilitation of attitude change if needed or desired
          (5)   Reduction of performance concerns
          (6)   Facilitation of effective communication and sexual functioning
          (7)   Examination of life-style issues
          (8)   Restructuring of sexual experience to facilitate effectiveness and pleasure

2.   Sexual health education should involve:
    a.   Identification of the nurse's and patient's value differences
    b.   A primary prevention approach
    c.   The view that sex education is a part of comprehensive education
    d.   Basic concepts for effective sex education, including:
          (1)   Sexuality is present at birth.
          (2)   Sexuality is inseparable from personal identity.
          (3)   Sexual thoughts and feelings are normal.
          (4)   Sexual behavior can be appropriate or inappropriate.
          (5)   There are appropriate and inappropriate times and places to act on sexual feelings.
          (6)   Sexuality encompasses one's total sense of self.
    e.   Correcting myths with the following facts:
          (1)   Most sexual dysfunction is due to sociocultural deprivation and ignorance.

    (2)   Masturbation is not harmful.
    (3)   Nymphomania does not exist.
    (4)   Menstrual flow is not harmful or dirty.
    (5)   Oral and anal sex are normal behaviors.
    (6)   Sexually promiscuous teens are not a product of excessive sex education.
    (7)   Most homosexuals do not molest children.
    (8)   Homosexuals are not sick and can control their behavior.
    (9)   Few homosexuals conform to stereotypes.
    (10)   Older adults continue to be sexual.
    (11)   Alcohol ingestion has not been proved to reduce inhibitions and enhance sexual enjoyment.

3. Intervening in sexual responses within the nurse–patient relationship encompasses:

  a.   Sexual responses of nurses to patients; important concepts include:
    (1)   Sexual responses are normal.
    (2)   Nurse should acknowledge feelings.
    (3)   Do not share personal information with patients.
    (4)   Avoid overinvolvement in patient's problems.
    (5)   Avoid discussing own feelings with patient.
    (6)   Seek consultation and support.

  b.   Sexual responses of patients to nurses; important concepts include:
    (1)   Patient seductiveness is a common occurrence.
    (2)   Let patient know behavior is unacceptable.
    (3)   Set limits on patient's behavior.
    (4)   Attempt to understand the sexual behavior.
    (5)   Assess meaning: attention-getting, reassurance of attractiveness, confused expression of gratitude.
    (6)   Explore meaning with patient.
    (7)   Define purpose of professional relationship.

4. Intervening in alteration of gender identity—transsexual responses—involves:

  a.   A therapist trained in human sexuality
  b.   Three stages:
    (1)   Thorough assessment
    (2)   Hormonal therapy
    (3)   Surgical reassignment
  c.   These prerequisites for treatment:
    (1)   Demonstrated sense of discomfort with own sex
    (2)   Wish to live as opposite sex
    (3)   Known to a professional therapist for 3 to 6 months
  d.   Usually at least 2 years for total treatment

5. Intervening in alterations in sexual orientation—maladaptive homosexual and bisexual responses—involves:
   a. Evaluating problems encountered by patients, including:
      (1) Difficulties from societal attitudes
      (2) Isolation from a support group
      (3) Pressure to choose between heterosexual and homosexual life-style
   b. Various steps in counseling:
      (1) Nurse's acceptance of patient
      (2) Patient's exploration of values and beliefs about homosexual people
      (3) Patient's exploration of internalized societal prejudices against homosexuality
      (4) Identification of coping behaviors: denial, confusion, sexual promiscuity
      (5) Discussion of patient's beliefs about homosexuality and bisexuality
      (6) Reading to discriminate myths from facts
      (7) Suggested actions for exploration (e.g., attend a homosexual social gathering)
6. Intervening in alterations of sexual functioning requires the nurse to have knowledge of treatment models and of credible sex therapists in the community; important models include:
   a. Masters and Johnson's model, involving:
      (1) Short-term education
      (2) Step-by-step instructions on physical aspects of sexual activity
      (3) Supportive psychotherapy
      (4) The belief that most sexual problems stem from ignorance, not psychiatric problems
      (5) Detailed sex history
      (6) Male–female therapeutic team for heterosexual couples
      (7) Round table discussion of therapists and patient couples
      (8) Sensate focus exercises
   b. Helen Singer Kaplan model, involving:
      (1) Psychodynamic principles
      (2) Conjoint therapeutic sessions
      (3) Behavioral tasks with psychodynamic insights
      (4) Single therapist
      (5) Extensive evaluation: psychiatric, sexual, marital, medical, family history
      (6) Therapy process with erotic tasks performed at home
      (7) Reactions processed during therapy sessions

D. **Evaluation**
1. The patient demonstrates increased awareness of precipitating stressor and ways to help reduce or eliminate these stressors.
2. The patient exhibits an increase in adaptive coping measures.
3. The patient reports an increased sense of well-being.
4. The patient reports restored or enhanced sexual functioning.
5. The patient reports satisfaction with treatment outcomes.

Bibliography

American Psychiatric Association (1987). *Diagnostic and statistical manual of mental disorders (DSM-III-R)* (3rd ed., revised). Washington, DC: Author.

Janosik, E. H., & Davies, E. L. (1987). *Psychiatric mental health nursing.* Boston: Jones & Bartlett.

Johnson, B. S. (1989). *Psychiatric-mental health nursing: Adaptation and growth* (2nd ed.). Philadelphia: J. B. Lippincott.

Stuart, G. W., & Sundeen, S. J. (1987). *Principles and practice of psychiatric nursing* (3rd ed.). St. Louis: C. V. Mosby.

Wilson, H. S., & Kneisl, C. R. (1988). *Psychiatric nursing* (3rd ed.). Menlo Park, CA: Addison-Wesley.

STUDY QUESTIONS

1. Which of the following factors is the most important requirement for nurses working at the basic level with patients in human sexuality?
   a. self-awareness and knowledge of normal sexual behavior
   b. knowledge about treatment approaches for conditions along the sexual health continuum
   c. ability to distinguish between normal and abnormal sexual behavior
   d. special training to use sex education or sex therapy approaches with patients

2. Bob, aged 18, has had 3 years of intermittent homosexual experience but continues to explain to staff that he isn't sure this is what he wants and flirts with young women on the unit. He reports sharply curtailing his sexual activity ever since he became aware of the possibility of contracting AIDS. The nurse caring for Bob should base initial nursing interventions on which of the following principles?
   a. Nurses provide social expectations and feedback for patients who are trying to modify their behavior.
   b. Nurses have a responsibility for teaching patients sexual health maintenance skills (e.g., sexual abstinence to prevent AIDS).
   c. Nurses can influence a patient's gender identity, which is continuously constructed throughout life.
   d. Nurses can help resolve a patient's sexual concerns by facilitating their clarification.

3. Ms. Abner, aged 20, complains of pain on intercourse and reports that she has been avoiding intercourse and feels angry with her partner. During assessment, which of the following actions would be of primary importance in determining the cause of dyspareunia?
   a. Explore her negative emotions toward her sexual partner.
   b. Ask about her relaxation level and degree of vaginal lubrication during sexual activity.
   c. Ask about her experience of orgasm.
   d. Perform a complete pelvic examination.

4. The nurse has been asked to provide a sex education program for high school students. Which of the following would *not* be an important consideration in conducting this type of health teaching?
   a. The nurse understands that her or his own values include intercourse only with marriage.
   b. Group discussion may reveal that some students believe sexual activity is appropriate or expected at their age.
   c. Negative consequences of sexual activity should be emphasized to prevent sexual promiscuity.
   d. Exploring students' values regarding sexual behavior helps them determine appropriate and inappropriate sexual behaviors.

5. Mr. Van Nort, who sustained a myocardial infarction 6 months ago, complains to his nurse that he can't "keep it up" during sexual activity. ("As soon as I try anything, I lose it.") Which of the following questions probably would be most helpful in clarifying his problem?
   a. "Are you having problems maintaining an erection?"
   b. "Are you having marital problems?"
   c. "When did your problem start?"
   d. "Are you afraid to have sex because of your heart attack?"

6. Ms. Lindros has just been admitted to a psychiatric unit with severe depression. When the nurse asks what prompted the hospitalization, Ms. Lindros sobs quietly, then says, "I haven't wanted sex for so long. I'm sure that's why our relationship is over." What would be the nurse's best response at this point?

a. "What exactly happened when he left?"
b. "You seem concerned about your sexual interest."
c. "This must have been an important relationship to you."
d. "Low sexual interest often is associated with depression."

7. Emily and Steve present with the complaint that intercourse does not last long enough because Steve ejaculates within seconds of penetration. Based on this information, the nurse could conclude that Steve is having a problem with which phase of the sexual response cycle?
a. orgasmic phase
b. arousal phase
c. interest or desire phase
d. resolution phase

8. A patient diagnosed with pedophilia has been admitted to the psychiatric unit for evaluation. The nursing staff learns that the patient has been sexually involved with several children from ages 8 to 10. Which would be the first step the staff needs to take in order to work effectively with this patient?
a. become familiar with the various theories explaining pedophilia
b. identify their own attitudes toward pedophilia
c. review the stages of sexual development
d. identify appropriate treatment approaches for pedophilia

9. Mr. Charles is taking Mellaril, a drug known to interfere with sexual arousal, inhibiting erections. When teaching Mr. Charles about the drug's side effects, the nurse should provide which of the following information?
a. Tell him to expect an erectile problem as a side effect.
b. Explain that his sexual desire likely will decrease.
c. Do not mention sexual side effects, to prevent anxiety from causing an erectile problem.

d. Explain that he should report any changes in his erections so medication adjustments can be considered.

10. A male patient exhibiting hypomanic behavior often makes sexually suggestive remarks to female staff members and one day tries to kiss a nurse. After telling the patient that this behavior is inappropriate, the nurse should respond to the patient with which of the following statements?
a. "It's normal for you to have sexual feelings."
b. "Let's talk about your feelings, so you can understand what you were trying to express."
c. "Let's discuss your sexual relationship in your marriage and what problems you may be having with it."
d. "It makes me uneasy when you make sexual advances toward me."

11. Helen, a 60-year-old widow, is undergoing her yearly physical, during which she expresses to the nurse that she has started dating seriously and has some concern about her ability to be sexually functional. Her physical examination reveals no abnormalities. Health history reveals that she is receiving estrogen replacement therapy and has not engaged in sexual activity for 10 years. The process of counseling Helen should include all of the following components *except*
a. teaching nondemand sexual activities to promote relaxation and anxiety reduction
b. providing information about normal physiologic changes due to the aging process
c. encouraging her view of herself as sexual
d. explaining that disuse often causes diminished sexual functioning

12. The nurse is working with an inpatient with a transsexual disorder who recently has started living as a member of the opposite sex. Appropriate outcome criteria for this nurse–patient relationship would include all of the following *except*

a. The patient will explore reactions and feelings about living in another gender role.
b. The patient will discuss feelings about the reactions experienced from others.
c. The patient will identify support persons to help during the change from one sex role to the other.
d. The patient will set the date for sex-change surgery.

ANSWER KEY

1. **Correct response: a**
   The basic level of intervention is based on the nurse's personal experiences. To be safe in working with a patient, the nurse needs to have self-awareness and some knowledge to prevent imposing personal values or giving inaccurate information.
   b, c, and d. This information is necessary for higher levels of intervention in sexual alterations, but self-awareness is the basic requirement for working in human sexuality.
   Knowledge/Health promotion/Assessment

2. **Correct response: d**
   This patient is exhibiting conflicts about his sexual orientation or pattern of sexual expression, indicating the need for exploration and clarification of his feelings about his homosexual behavior.
   a. This principle assumes that the nurse should promote social expectations and provide feedback for what the nurse decides is desired behavior, rather than what the patient chooses. This approach would limit the patient's exploration and self-understanding.
   b. The patient seems to be expressing a conflict between a homosexual and a heterosexual orientation as a priority need. Methods to prevent AIDS would need to be addressed at some point, being careful to avoid negativism about homosexuality.
   c. Gender identity refers to one's personal sense of being male or female. A disorder in gender identity is transsexualism, which is not this patient's problem. Although gender identity may influence sexual orientation, it is not the same as sexual orientation.
   Analysis/Psychosocial/Implementation

3. **Correct response: d**

In most cases, dyspareunia stems from physiologic conditions.
   a. Negative emotions usually are a result of dyspareunia, rather than a cause.
   b and c. Tension and lack of lubrication are common causes of dyspareunia, and inhibited orgasm can cause uncomfortable congestion in the genital area and lower back. However, without the physical examination, the validity of any of these causes could not be trusted.
   Analysis/Health promotion/Assessment

4. **Correct response: c**
   There is no evidence to indicate that sex education promotes promiscuity. Adolescents could respond negatively if negative consequences are introduced as threats.
   a. The nurse's values need to be clearly identified and efforts made to avoid value impositions during teaching.
   b. It is important for patients or students to explore and understand their own values about sexuality.
   d. Students need exploration and guidance in determining appropriate sexual behaviors.
   Application/Health promotion/Planning

5. **Correct response: a**
   The phase of the sexual response cycle following interest or desire is arousal (involving erection in men). The nurse needs to clarify the sexual problem as presented by the patient before moving to other areas of assessment.
   b. This question focuses away from the sexual problem presented and may be used to protect the nurse from anxiety about sexuality.
   c. This question would be appropriate in assessment (sex problem history) but is inappropriately timed here. It should be asked after the problem is clarified.

d. Although fear could be a possible cause of the problem, the problem is not yet sufficiently clarified for exploration of its origins or causes.

Application/Psychosocial/Assessment

6. **Correct response: c**

The patient did not use a specific gender when referring to her relationship, indicating that she could be lesbian. The nurse needs to be aware of all possibilities of sexual orientation at this time in the assessment and must avoid inadvertent value imposition. This is the most sensitive nonjudgmental nursing response to a patient who may be testing to see if she can safely reveal her lesbian sexual orientation.

   a. This response assumes the gender of the partner without knowing the patient's orientation and represents value imposition on the nurse's part.

   b. The sexual interest problem is secondary to the patient's obvious grief at this moment. Responses need to be based on a holistic as well as sexual assessment.

   d. This response provides correct information at an inappropriate time (*i.e.*, during early assessment without adequate information or a nursing diagnosis).

Analysis/Psychosocial/Assessment

7. **Correct response: a**

Ejaculation occurs in the orgasmic phase, and Steve suffers premature ejaculation.

   b. Erectile problems would involve arousal phase disorders.

   c. There is no indication that he is experiencing problems with sexual desire.

   d. The primary problem described does not involve the resolution phase.

Knowledge/Psychosocial/Analysis (Dx)

8. **Correct response: b**

Sexual molestation of children is socially unacceptable; nurses' negative attitudes and biases need to be confronted through the self-awareness process in the preinteraction stage. This helps prevent personal feelings from interfering with the nurse's understanding of the condition and with therapeutic intervention.

   a, c, and d. These issues are secondary to being aware of one's own values, attitudes, and biases.

Comprehension/Health promotion/Analysis (Dx)

9. **Correct response: d**

Patients have a right to information about drug side effects. Patients often discontinue medication to avoid or correct sexual side effects and are less likely to do that if health professionals offer assistance with sexual issues. Patients generally will not raise sexual issues unless health professionals give permission by raising the issue first.

   a. This response promotes the expectation of a sexual problem, which can create performance anxiety and lead to erectile failure.

   b. Impaired sexual desire most likely would be secondary to the erectile dysfunction.

   c. This response does not allow discussion of this sensitive issue. It likely reflects the nurse's avoidance of uncomfortable feelings.

Application/Psychosocial/Implementation

10. **Correct response: b**

Identifying the meaning of the patient's behavior promotes understanding and helps the patient gain self-control through verbal expression of the underlying feelings.

   a. Although this is a correct statement, it is not appropriate for this situation. The nurse would be making an assumption that the patient's behavior was sexually motivated, when it may not have been. The statement could also reinforce inappropriate behavior.

c. This issue may be important later, but it would not be a priority response at this time.

d. This response addresses the nurse's feelings rather than the patient's behavior and feelings, which would distract from the patient's learning.

Application/Health promotion/Implementation

11. **Correct response: d**

This intervention would discourage the interest she has shown and would be more likely to inhibit her than to develop her sexual ability. Even though this information is accurate, there must be a therapeutic purpose in providing it to the patient.

a. Nondemand sexual activities allow pleasurable, sexually stimulating touch without the threat of intercourse, leading to anxiety reduction and confidence building.

b. This action would help the patient prepare for differences in the sexual experience as compared with her earlier experiences.

c. By encouraging the patient to view herself as a sexual being, the nurse can help the patient avoid incorporating the myth of the aging person as asexual into her personal belief system.

Analysis/Health promotion/Implementation

12. **Correct response: d**

Unless the nurse is a certified sex therapist, this would not be an expected outcome from nursing care of this patient.

a, b, and c. These are all areas that need to be explored by the patient, which the nurse could facilitate by using therapeutic listening skills.

Application/Psychosocial/Evaluation

Substance Abuse Disorders

8

I. Overview

A. Definitions

1. Substances: alcohol, prescription drugs, over-the-counter medications, and illicit drugs
2. Abuse: use of a chemical substance for purposes other than medical treatment, especially with resulting life situation problems
3. Tolerance: the need for increasingly large doses of a substance in
   order to produce effects previously achieved by smaller doses
4. Addiction: a group of behavioral and physical symptoms indicating impaired control of substances; psychoactive dependence
   a. Physical dependence: the body's biologic need for a sub-
      stance

      b.   Psychologic dependence: craving for the subjective effect of a substance

B.   **Incidence**

1.   Substance abuse affects people of all ages, cultural groups, and socioeconomic classes.

2.   About one in 10 American workers is a substance abuser.

3.   Almost one half of all families in the United States have problems with substances.

4.   About one in five nurses is a substance abuser.

5.   Alcohol is the most commonly abused substance; over 10 million people in the United States are alcoholics.

6.   Over 3 million teenagers are problem drinkers.

7.   An estimated 4 million people in the United States are cocaine abusers.

C.   **Commonly abused substances**

1.   Central nervous system (CNS) depressants, which can cause depression of the respiratory system, include:
    a.   Alcohol
    b.   Sedative (e.g., secobarbital), hypnotic (e.g., Quaalude), and antianxiety (e.g., diazepam) drugs
    c.   Opioids (e.g., Demerol, codeine, heroin)

2.   CNS stimulants promote psychologic dependence, which tends to be more powerful than the physical dependence; types include:
    a.   Amphetamines (e.g., Dexedrine)
    b.   Cocaine

3.   Mind-altering substances, which promote psychologic dependence, include:
    a.   Hallucinogens (e.g., LSD)
    b.   Cannabis (marijuana, hashish)
    c.   Phencyclidine (PCP or angel dust)

4.   Polysubstance abuse involves concurrent abuse of two or more substances (e.g., heroin and cocaine, marijuana and cocaine, alcohol and barbiturates).

D.   **Etiology of substance abuse**

1.   Biologic factors associated with substance abuse include:
    a.   Familial (possibly genetic) tendency
    b.   Metabolic factors (e.g., ethanol metabolized more efficiently, with less effect in some alcoholics)

2.   Psychologic factors include:
    a.   Codependent personality
    b.   Insecurity
    c.   Maladaptive coping skills

3.   Sociologic factors include:
    a.   Enmeshed (overly dependent) family relationships

      b.   Dysfunctional family communication

      c.   Peer pressure

      d.   Easy access to substances

      e.   Societal ambivalence about substance use

      f.   Societal messages that medicine solves all problems

E. **Characteristics of substance abuse and dependence (addiction)**

    1.   Substance abuse involves at least one of the following behaviors for at least 1 month's duration:

      a.   Continues use of a substance despite awareness of the problems it produces or exacerbates

      b.   Continues use of substance under dangerous situations

      c.   Uses defense mechanisms of denial, rationalization, and projection concerning substances, use, and results

    2.   Substance dependence involves any three of the following behaviors for more than 1 month's duration:

      a.   Consumes more than is intended and over a longer time period than intended

      b.   Is unable to control excessive use of the substance

      c.   Spends a great amount of time getting, taking, and recovering from the substance

      d.   Is unable to fulfill responsibilities because of intoxication or withdrawal symptoms

      e.   Reduces former activities; life revolves around substance use

      f.   Experiences biopsychosocial problems from substance use

      g.   Develops tolerance; needs more of the substance to produce intoxication or a high

      h.   Experiences withdrawal with discontinued or reduced use of the substance

      i.   Takes the substance to prevent withdrawal symptoms

II. **Types of substance abuse**

  A.   Alcoholism

    1.   Route of ingestion: oral

    2.   Typical users: adults, teens

    3.   Common related dangers include:

      a.   Car accidents, physical injury

      b.   Malnutrition

      c.   Medical problems (e.g., hepatitis, cirrhosis, gastritis)

      d.   Suicide

      e.   Fetal alcohol syndrome

  B.   Sedative-hypnotic, antianxiety drug abuse

    1.   Route of ingestion: oral or parenteral

    2.   Typical users: middle-class, middle-aged women, teens, young adults

    3.   Related dangers include:

a. CNS depression

b. Overdose, death especially with alcohol

C. **Opioid abuse**

1. Route of ingestion: oral, intravenous, intramuscular, subcutaneous, smoking, nasal inhalation
2. Typical users: teens, young adults
3. Related dangers include:
    a. Malnutrition
    b. Hepatitis and other infections
    c. Shock, respiratory depression
    d. Acquired immune deficiency syndrome (AIDS)
    e. Death

D. **Amphetamine abuse**

1. Route of ingestion: oral, intravenous
2. Typical users: teens, young adults
3. Related dangers include:
    a. Malnutrition
    b. Convulsions
    c. Depression
    d. Suicide

E. **Cocaine abuse**

1. Route of ingestion: nasal inhalation, subcutaneous injection, smoking
2. Typical users: teens, young adults
3. Related dangers include:
    a. Dizziness
    b. Fever
    c. Depression
    d. Convulsions, cardiac or respiratory arrest, death

F. **Mind-altering substance (e.g., marijuana) abuse**

1. Route of ingestion: smoking, oral
2. Typical users: teens, young adults
3. Related dangers include:
    a. Impaired judgment and psychomotor skills (e.g., driving)
    b. Lack of motivation, apathy
    c. Lung problems
    d. Panic reaction

III. **Nursing process in substance abuse**

A. **Assessment**

1. Common assessment findings in alcohol dependence include:
    a. Physiologic responses
        (1) Development of tolerance
        (2) Hangovers: headache, gastric problems (nausea, vomiting, gastritis), fatigue, sweating

(3) Blackouts: inability to recall events that occurred while intoxicated

(4) Loss of consciousness

(5) Withdrawal, resulting from discontinuation of drinking; characterized by anxiety, tremulousness, disorientation, and auditory hallucinations; can last up to a week

(6) Delirium tremens, characterized by increased intensity of symptoms in withdrawal and occurring 48 to 72 hours after the last drink; involves more pronounced disorientation, anxiousness, tremulousness, anorexia, insomnia, tachycardia, vomiting, visual hallucinations, seizures

(7) Damage to internal organs: irritation of the esophagus, gastritis, cirrhosis of the liver, fatty liver, pancreatitis, thiamine deficiency, hepatitis

(8) Fetal alcohol syndrome: a condition affecting infants born to alcoholic mothers involving intellectual deficits, physical abnormalities, and signs of alcohol dependence and requiring withdrawal from alcohol

b. Behavioral responses
    (1) Loudness, verbosity, slurred speech
    (2) Aggressiveness
    (3) Reduced inhibitions
    (4) Concealment of drinking from significant others
    (5) Drinking in the morning
    (6) Failure to fulfill social, occupational, and familial responsibilities
    (7) Accident proneness; trouble with the law (e.g., driving under the influence of alcohol)

c. Cognitive responses
    (1) Short attention span
    (2) Reduced concentration and alertness
    (3) Poor recall
    (4) Poor judgment and insight

d. Affective responses
    (1) Mood ranging from happy to sad to irritable
    (2) Emotional lability

e. Potentiated effects of barbiturates, tranquilizers, narcotics, and sleeping pills—commonly combined in suicide attempts

2. Assessment findings in barbiturate dependence (somewhat similar to those in alcohol dependence) include:

a. Physiologic responses
    (1) During withdrawal, elevated temperature and

blood pressure, postural hypotension, insomnia, anorexia, tremors, seizures, possible respiratory failure
- (2) Loss of consciousness
- (3) Signs of dependence in infants born to mothers dependent on barbiturates; withdrawal is necessary
  b. Behavioral responses
    - (1) Reduced inhibitions
    - (2) Unsteady gait, poor motor coordination
    - (3) Slurred speech
    - (4) Verbosity
    - (5) Doctor-shopping for prescriptions
  c. Cognitive responses
    - (1) Poor judgment and insight
    - (2) Decreased alertness
    - (3) Poor attention span
    - (4) Poor recall
  d. Affective responses
    - (1) Mood ranging from initial happiness to hostility, irritability, agitation, and apprehension
    - (2) Emotional lability
3. Signs of opioid dependence include:
  a. Physiologic responses
    - (1) Constricted pupils
    - (2) Reduced responsiveness to pain
    - (3) Nausea and vomiting
    - (4) Withdrawal symptoms: muscle aches, nausea and vomiting, abdominal cramping, decreased appetite, sweating, runny nose, fever, diarrhea, restlessness, fatigue
    - (5) Signs of dependence in infants born to mothers dependent on opioids; safe withdrawal is needed
    - (6) In some cases, signs and symptoms of infection (hepatitis, AIDS) related to the use of dirty needles and other drug paraphernalia
  b. Behavioral responses
    - (1) Drowsiness
    - (2) Slurred speech
    - (3) Poor motor coordination
    - (4) Disinterest in surroundings
    - (5) Use of illegal means to acquire substance
  c. Cognitive responses
    - (1) Poor concentration
    - (2) Poor recall
    - (3) Poor judgment and insight

      d.   Affective responses
            (1)   Mood swings from euphoria to depression
            (2)   Apathy

4. Manifestations of amphetamine and cocaine dependence can include:
      a.   Physiologic responses
            (1)   Insomnia
            (2)   Anorexia, weight loss
            (3)   Tachycardia
            (4)   Hypertension
            (5)   Seizures
            (6)   Hyperthermia
            (7)   Respiratory arrest
            (8)   In infants born to mothers dependent on cocaine, irritability and possibly seizures and brain damage
      b.   Behavioral responses
            (1)   Hyperactivity
            (2)   Hypervigilance
            (3)   Delusions and hallucinations similar to those found in paranoid schizophrenia
      c.   Cognitive responses
            (1)   Grandiose ideations
            (2)   Poor judgment
            (3)   Poor concentration
            (4)   Poor attention span
            (5)   Poor recall
      d.   Affective responses
            (1)   Euphoria followed by dysphoria, characterized by anhedonia, social isolation, reduced energy
            (2)   Anxiousness
            (3)   Agitation
            (4)   Continuation of substance use related to strong psychologic desire
            (5)   In withdrawal, psychologic depression (which can lead to suicide), excessive eating and sleeping, muscle aches, and generalized discomfort

5. Effects of hallucinogen dependence may include:
      a.   Physiologic responses
            (1)   Heightened sensory experiences
            (2)   Hallucinations
      b.   Behavioral responses
            (1)   Unpredictable behavior
            (2)   Self-destructive behavior
      c.   Cognitive responses
            (1)   Poor judgment
            (2)   Delusions

                    (3)   "Bad trips" that may mimic schizophrenia
        d.   Affective responses
              (1)   Anxiety
              (2)   Fear

6. Manifestations of cannabis dependence may include:
    a. Physiologic responses
        (1) Reduced reflex timing
        (2) Conjunctival redness
    b. Behavioral responses: reduced inhibition
    c. Cognitive responses
        (1) Poor attention span
        (2) Poor recall
    d. Affective responses
        (1) Euphoria followed by apathy, irritability
        (2) Reduced motivation

7. Phencyclidine dependence may be marked by:
    a. Physiologic responses
        (1) Hypertension
        (2) Nausea and vomiting
        (3) Ataxia
        (4) Seizures
        (5) Decreased pain response
    b. Behavioral responses
        (1) Extreme violent behavior followed by unresponsiveness
        (2) Bizarre behavior that can mimic paranoid schizophrenia
    c. Cognitive responses
        (1) Poor judgment
        (2) Impaired reality testing
    d. Affective responses
        (1) Agitation
        (2) Confusion

8. Other areas to assess include:
    a. Amount and purity of substance used
    b. Frequency of use (daily, weekend, recreational use)
    c. Method of use (smoking and intravenous use lead to abuse and dependence quicker than does oral use)
    d. Last dose
    e. The method of obtaining it (e.g., prescription, prostitution, stealing)
    f. The effects of not having the substance
    g. If an overdose, was it intentional
    h. Biopsychosocial consequences of use
    i. Stressors in the person's life
    j. Defense mechanisms employed

k.   Prior treatments and outcomes
l.   Support systems (familial, social, and financial)
m.   Patient's self-perception, level of self-esteem
n.   Manipulative behavior
B. Analysis and nursing diagnoses
1.   The nurse should identify the substance used and its effects on the person and his or her significant others.
2.   Pertinent North American Nursing Diagnosis Association (NANDA) nursing diagnoses may include:
a.   Sensory-Perceptual Alteration
(1)   Related to effect of substance
(2)   Related to withdrawal symptoms
b.   Altered Thought Processes
(1)   Related to effect of substance
(2)   Related to psychologic dependence
c.   Ineffective Individual Coping
(1)   Related to continuous use of substance
(2)   Related to limited social and assertiveness skills
d.   Disturbance in Self-Concept
(1)   Related to inability to handle feelings
(2)   Related to the use of denial and other defense mechanisms to maintain substance use
(3)   Related to inability to recognize positive qualities
C. Planning and implementation
1.   Interventions for promoting withdrawal from substances include:
a.   Observing and monitoring patient's vital signs and symptoms
b.   Providing a safe environment void of illicit substance use; reducing unnecessary stimuli and risk of harm
c.   Stabilizing patient to his optimal level of functioning
d.   Providing support and reassurance
e.   Promoting adequate nutrition
f.   Following physician's orders for detoxification
2.   Assist the patient to practice abstinence by:
a.   Establishing mutually agreed-upon goals that are clearly stated and that delineate the patient's responsibilities
b.   Providing education focusing on the biopsychosocial symptoms and consequences of substance abuse (the progressive chronic course of dependency, the phenomenon of recidivism, the symptoms and treatment, defense mechanisms typically employed, community resources available to the patient); educating the patient and his or her significant others
c.   Avoiding judgmental behavior; being aware of biases that will affect treatment

        d.   Avoiding rejecting or belittling the patient

        e.   Not playing the role of enabler

  3.   Help the patient understand the dynamics of substance dependence behavior.

        a.   Establish a therapeutic relationship in which the patient is respected.

        b.   Assist patient to express anger constructively (to label his or her feelings).

        c.   Assist patient to examine his or her maladaptive behavior and its meaning.

        d.   Assist patient to recognize his or her strengths; reinforce patient's strengths.

        e.   Assist patient to recognize his or her defense mechanisms and the role they play in maintaining his dependence.

        f.   Encourage participation in individual, group, or family therapy as well as self-help groups.

        g.   Teach assertive skills and adaptive social skills.

D. **Evaluation**

  1.   The patient reports discontinued use of harmful substances.

  2.   The patient demonstrates reduced or absent physiologic, behavioral, cognitive, and affective manifestations of substance dependence.

  3.   The patient (and family members, if applicable) reports improved family, social, and occupational functioning.

Bibliography

Janosik, E. H., & Davies, E. L. (1987). *Psychiatric mental health nursing.* Boston: Jones & Bartlett.

Johnson, B. S. (1989). *Psychiatric-mental health nursing: Adaptation and growth* (2nd ed.). Philadelphia: J. B. Lippincott.

Johnson, G., & Hannah, K. (1987). *Pharmacology and the nursing process* (2nd ed.). Philadelphia: W. B. Saunders.

Rodman, M., & Karch, A. (1985). *Pharmacology and drug therapy in Nursing* (3rd ed.). Philadelphia: J. B. Lippincott.

Stuart, G. W., & Sundeen, S. J. (1987). *Principles and practice of psychiatric nursing* (3rd ed.). St. Louis: C. V. Mosby.

Wilson, H. S., & Kneisl, C. R. (1988). *Psychiatric nursing* (3rd ed.). Menlo Park, CA: Addison-Wesley.

STUDY QUESTIONS

1. What is the difference between substance dependence and substance abuse?
   a. Substance dependence is less severe than substance abuse.
   b. Substance dependence is characterized by withdrawal, whereas substance abuse is not.
   c. Substance dependence involves continued use of the substance for at least 1 month; substance abuse does not.
   d. Substance dependence is not characterized by increased tolerance, whereas substance abuse is.

2. Ms. Smith, a 25-year-old registered nurse, entered treatment after she was fired from her job because of theft of morphine. She tells the nurse that she was framed. The nurse responds, ''That kind of thing happens often.'' This response would be
   a. helpful, because it provides support for Ms. Smith
   b. not helpful because it increases stress
   c. helpful because it paves the way for a therapeutic relationship
   d. not helpful because it supports Ms. Smith's defenses

3. Which of the following nursing diagnoses likely would be appropriate for Ms. Smith?
   a. Impaired Verbal Communication
   b. Sensory-Perceptual Alteration
   c. Knowledge Deficit
   d. Impaired Physical Immobility

4. The initial plan of care for Ms. Smith should involve
   a. making appropriate outpatient referrals
   b. providing assertiveness training
   c. teaching about the risk of losing her nursing license
   d. promoting a safe environment devoid of illicit substance use

5. Defense mechanisms commonly associated with substance dependence include
   a. repression and reaction formation
   b. denial and projection
   c. rationalization and sublimation
   d. regression and displacement

6. Mrs. Jones, a high school teacher, reports a need to drink 4 to 5 glasses of wine after work and to take a couple of sleeping pills before bedtime. She also reports taking diazepam (Valium) frequently while at school to ''calm my nerves.'' In addition, she chain smokes. She is concerned because she is experiencing an inability to concentrate and to attend to her classes as well as a reduction in the ability to censor her behavior. She does not perceive her current status of substance use as being related to her concerns. The nurse should recognize that Mrs. Jones has a
   a. polysubstance dependence because of equal dependence on three substances
   b. polysubstance dependence because of equal dependence on four substances
   c. alcohol dependence because her primary problem is alcohol
   d. benzodiazepine dependence because her primary problem is benzodiazepine use

7. The symptoms reported by Mrs. Jones are typical of
   a. barbiturate dependence
   b. hypnotic dependence
   c. CNS depression
   d. antianxiety agent dependence

8. The nurse should tell Mrs. Jones that her substance use constitutes a primary danger because it can lead to
   a. loss of employment
   b. loss of respect from her students and colleagues
   c. lethal overdose
   d. reduced self-esteem

9. The nurse's initial plan should be to assist Mrs. Jones to
   a. recognize her depression

b. develop healthy coping strategies

c. understand the dynamics of substance dependence

d. become cognizant of the biopsychosocial consequences of her substance dependence

10. Mrs. Jones recognizes the need to discontinue her substance use. The nurse recommends

   a. Alcoholics Anonymous
   b. inpatient treatment
   c. family therapy
   d. crisis intervention

11. Ann, a slightly obese young woman, was admitted to a psychiatric unit after exhibiting bizarre, suspicious behavior. She was extremely agitated but was able to tell the nurse that she had been taking pills to help her lose weight. Ann was most likely taking

   a. LSD
   b. barbiturates
   c. phencyclidine
   d. amphetamines

12. The nurse would expect Ann's behavior to be extremely unpredictable and to vacillate between extreme violence and nonresponsiveness if she had taken

   a. marijuana
   b. barbiturates
   c. phencyclidine
   d. amphetamines

13. The nurse's plans include minimizing Ann's withdrawal. This plan is necessary because withdrawal

   a. results in delirium tremens
   b. can be life-threatening
   c. is psychologically uncomfortable
   d. mimics flu symptoms

14. The nurse would evaluate Ann's progress positively if Ann made which of the following statements?

   a. "I'm ready for discharge."
   b. "I don't need to be here with these crazy people."
   c. "I only used the pills to lose weight."
   d. "Taking those pills got out of control."

ANSWER KEY

1. *Correct response: b*
   Substance dependence is characterized by withdrawal and increased tolerance and is more severe than substance abuse. Both substance dependence and abuse have durations of at least 1 month.
   a, c, and d. These responses are all inaccurate descriptions.
   Comprehension/Physiologic/Analysis (Dx)

2. *Correct response: d*
   This statement would not be helpful because it would fail to assist Ms. Smith in recognizing her defense mechanisms and how these defenses foster her continued substance use.
   a and c. These responses would support Ms. Smith's defenses and therefore are nontherapeutic.
   b. This statement would remove any pressure for Ms. Smith to begin the change process.
   Analysis/Psychosocial/Implementation

3. *Correct response: c*
   From the information presented in this situation, it is apparent that Ms. Smith demonstrates impaired judgment and impaired insight.
   a, b, and d. Not enough information is provided to justify a diagnosis of impaired communication, altered sensory perception, or impaired physical mobility.
   Application/Psychosocial/Analysis (Dx)

4. *Correct response: d*
   It is not uncommon for patients in treatment programs to try to elicit substances.
   a, b, and c. These options may be necessary for intermediate or long-term planning.
   Application/Psychosocial/Planning

5. *Correct response: b*
   Defenses commonly employed in sub-

stance dependence include denial, projection, and rationalization.
   a, c, and d. Repression, reaction formation, sublimation, regression, and displacement are not commonly used in substance dependence.
   Knowledge/Psychosocial/Assessment

6. *Correct response: a*
   Polysubstance dependence is characterized by equal dependence on at least three substances, excluding nicotine.
   b. Cigarette smoking is not included in polysubstance dependence.
   c and d. Neither benzodiazepines nor alcohol alone is her primary problem.
   Analysis/Psychosocial/Analysis (Dx)

7. *Correct response: c*
   The substances Mrs. Jones is using all belong to the CNS depressant category. Her symptoms are typical for this category of substances.
   a, b and d. These substances are all subsumed under the CNS depressant category.
   Application/Psychosocial/Analysis (Dx)

8. *Correct response: c*
   Alcohol, sleeping pills, and minor tranquilizers enhance the depressive quality of each other, thus making the combination much more potent than the single substance. This potentiating effect can be dangerous and can inadvertently lead to an overdose.
   a, b, and d. Even though these problems may result from Mrs. Jones' polysubstance dependence, they don't constitute the primary danger.
   Application/Health promotion/ Implementation

9. *Correct response: d*
   Mrs. Jones is denying any association

126

between her concerns and her substance use. Providing Mrs. Jones with didactic information regarding the biopsychosocial consequences of her polysubstance dependence may assist Mrs. Jones in making this association.

    a. There is no indication of Mrs. Jones being depressed.

    b and c. These are long-term and intermediate plans, respectively.

Application/Health promotion/Planning

10. *Correct response: b*
Inpatient treatment would provide a complete medical workup, detoxification if needed, multiple treatment approaches (e.g., group and individual therapy, self-help groups), and a safe, structured milieu.

    a, c, and d. None of these options fully addresses Mrs. Jones' problem.

Application/Health promotion/Evaluation

11. *Correct response: d*
Amphetamines sometimes are used to induce weight loss, which produces the side effects described in the scenario.

    a and c. Although the side effects of these substances can be similar to the ones described in this situation, neither is taken to promote weight loss.

    b. This CNS depressant generally does not induce bizarre, suspicious behavior.

Application/Psychosocial/Analysis (Dx)

12. *Correct response: c*
Persons taking phencyclidine display unpredictable behavior, vacillating between nonresponsiveness and violence. These persons are considered dangerous to themselves and to others.

    a, b, and d. None of these substances involves the same degree of dangerousness (violence) as phencyclidine.

Application/Psychosocial/Analysis (Dx)

13. *Correct response: c*
Amphetamine dependence results in a strong psychologic craving, and withdrawal is characterized by a depressive episode.

    a, b, and d. These withdrawal symptoms are typically found in alcohol, barbiturate, and heroin dependence, respectively.

Application/Safe care/Planning

14. *Correct response: d*
This response gives an indication that Ann has some understanding of the dynamics of substance dependence.

    a, b, and c. These responses demonstrate a lack of insight.

Application/Psychosocial/Evaluation

Family Violence

I. Overview

A. Definitions

1. Violence: physical force exerted for the purpose of violating, damaging, or abusing; abusive or unjust exercise of power often resulting in physical injury
2. Abuse: to use wrongly or improperly; to hurt or injure by maltreatment (can be physical or psychologic)
3. Offender: person who perpetrates abuse or violence on another
4. Victim: person who is the scapegoat, target, recipient of abuse or violence

B. Incidence

1. Family violence occurs across many boundaries, including:
   a. All socioeconomic levels
   b. Both genders
   c. All ages
   d. Every geographic area

        e.   Every racial, religious, educational, and occupational background

2. Prevalence is difficult to determine because incidents are underreported (an estimated 10 to 20 unreported cases for each reported case).
3. In three of five families, a child suffers physical abuse by an adult.
4. Two million cases of female and male violence each are reported annually.
5. One in seven married women report marital rape. One in six couples will experience abuse each year.
6. One to two million cases of elderly abuse occur each year.
7. Any member of a dysfunctional family is at risk for involvement in violence.

C. Common acts of abuse or violence
1. Physical injury (minor to lethal)
2. Threats of physical harm, usually to intimidate and manipulate
3. Inappropriate sexual activity
   a. Behavior ranging from sexually stimulating talk or actions to inappropriate touching or intercourse; may include perverse sexual behaviors including rape
   b. Incest: sexual behavior between relatives
4. Exposing family members to illegal activity, including prostitution or substance abuse involvement
5. Neglect of family member's person and basic needs:
   a. Food
   b. Water
   c. Warmth
   d. Cleanliness
   e. Health care, including preventive care
   f. Social contact
   g. For children, educational and supervision requirements
6. Undermining personal needs for security:
   a. Threats of abandonment (including suicide)
   b. Institutionalization
   c. Eviction
   d. Gross instability of environment
7. Undermining development and maintenance of self-esteem:
   a. Devaluation
   b. Harsh or unrealistic criticism
   c. Unrealistic or unreasonable expectations
8. Undermining development and maintenance of a sense of self and personal boundaries:
   a. Lack of interpersonal validation and other feedback
   b. Inconsistency in interactions

D. Etiology
1. No single cause accounts for family violence; various theories attempt to explain facets of the problem.

2. Systems theory posits that violence occurs as a result of tension produced by a dysfunctional family system; sources of this tension can include:
    a. Individual family member
    b. System interaction
    c. Environment
    d. Society
3. Structural theories involve such problems as unclear boundaries and enmeshment of individuals and roles.
4. Social learning theory explains that violence is a learned behavior.
5. Environment-stress theory states that social attitudes and pressures influence both abuser and victim.
6. Psychodynamic theories link family violence to personal histories and conflicts influencing lack of ego strengths, impulse controls, and nurturing capacities. (Abusers commonly have a history of being abused themselves.)
7. Epidemiologic theories propose that various risk factors increase the potential for violence, including:
    a. Motivation to abuse (immaturity, need to control, mental illness, conflicts)
    b. Overcoming internal factors inhibiting abuse (e.g., impaired reality testing, substance abuse)
    c. Overcoming external factors inhibiting abuse (e.g., environment conducive to tension, overstimulation)
    d. Overcoming a person's resistance (e.g., very young, naive or uninformed, in need of affection, coerced)
E. **Characteristics of dysfunctional family leading to abuse or violence**
    1. Closed system with poor coping capacities
        a. Family boundaries are rigid or chaotic and undifferentiated.
        b. Roles are stereotypic and stifling; there are traditional sex roles and a strong power differential between parent(s) and children.
        c. Rules are inflexible; there is authoritarian behavior and unreasonable expectations.
        d. Relationships emphasize control and power differentials; dependence and enmeshment may occur.
        e. Achievement and maintenance of trust is difficult, leading to secrecy and isolation.
        f. Communication patterns are dysfunctional (e.g., denial and conflict avoidance, double-bind patterns, conditional loving, poor impulse control over emotions, rationalization of abuse or violence).
        g. Stresses and pressures often exist, placing overwhelming demands on those with poor coping capacities (e.g., financial insecurity, personal insecurity or poor character development, psychopathology, substance abuse).

      h.   Problem-solving strategies are impaired.

2.   Predictable characteristics of members of abusive or violent families
    a.   Adults may have personal histories of being abused or of violent behavior.
    b.   Adults may be immature or lacking in effective coping capacities.
    c.   One or more adults may be authoritarian and rigid in expectations.

3.   Male adults are the most frequent perpetrators of child sexual abuse and spouse abuse; characteristics of an abusive male may include:
    a.   Controlling and dominating
    b.   Poor self-esteem, triggering a need to bolster self-esteem through enforcing submission and dependence
    c.   High frustration level, with family members becoming targets of displaced frustration and aggression

4.   An abusive male may seek inappropriate sexual gratification to act out personal issues and dysfunction in relationship with spouse or partner.

5.   Adult females are the most frequent violent perpetrators of child physical abuse and the most frequent abusers of the elderly; some characteristics of female abusers include:
    a.   May abuse as outlet for frustration and anger related to stress and unmet needs
    b.   May respond with violence after history of victim behavior
    c.   Often financially and emotionally dependent on spouse or partner
    d.   Unsuccessfully adopts submissive, passive role in attempt to avoid abuse
    e.   May not recognize or question marital rape
    f.   May accept personal abuse to protect another family member
    g.   May rationalize abuse ("He was drunk," "He apologized") and avoid changing situation or pressing charges

6.   Children are most often the victims but also can be the perpetrator of abuse or violence. Male and female victim incidence is equal, with female children more often victimized sexually. Brother–brother violence is the most common form of sibling abuse.

7.   Elderly adults may be victims and may have been abusers when younger; common characteristics include:
    a.   Usually the parents of their abusers
    b.   Usually physically or mentally impaired
    c.   May place financial, emotional, time, and physical stresses on family and primary caretakers, exceeding resources to meet their needs

        d.   May be aggressive or submissive, creating emotional reaction in abuser

        e.   May be unwilling or unable to report abuse

II.   Types of abuse or violence

   A. **Physical**

       1. Beating, hitting, cutting, shooting, burning, raping

       2. Withholding personal care, basic needs

       3. Lack of supervision

       4. Inadequate environment

   B. **Psychologic**

       1. Verbal assault and threats

       2. Sarcasm, humiliation, devaluing, criticism, or withdrawal and silence

       3. Disturbed, inconsistent communication patterns

   C. **Material**

       1. Theft of money or property

       2. Misuse of money or property

   D. **Social**

       1. Violation of rights (shelter, family and friends, social activities)

       2. Isolation resulting from fear or embarrassment of acknowledging abuse or violence to others

   E. **Sexual**

       1. Pressured or forced sexual activity

       2. Overt inappropriate sexual behavior (e.g., exposure of genitals, provocative language)

III. Nursing process in family violence

   A. **Assessment**

       1. Routine recognition of predisposing factors involves evaluating the family system for:

          a.   Stresses on family unit, such as:

             (1)   Financial difficulty

             (2)   Need for sense of worth in community

             (3)   Family member(s) placing high demands for time, supervision, care

             (4)   Inadequate housing, food, warmth, health care

             (5)   Inadequate environment (poor housing, crowding)

             (6)   Conflict between family, extended family, community

             (7)   Frustration (often chronic) resulting from attempts to function

             (8)   Acute situational crisis

          b.   Impaired or reduced adaptive capacities, including:

             (1)   History of disorganized functioning (going from crisis to crisis)

        (2)   Lack of knowledge about human development, aspects of healthy relationships, available options

        (3)   Lack of knowledge about problem-solving process

        (4)   Inadequate resources or support for family's attempts to cope

c.   Family style interfering with healthy functioning, such as:

        (1)   Closed system, isolation

        (2)   Denial and maintenance of family secrets maintained

        (3)   Inability to tolerate stress, anger

        (4)   Impaired communication patterns

        (5)   Poor impulse control, inability to delay gratification

        (6)   Lack of long-term planning

d.   Family member(s) unable to support healthy functioning of family system, marked by:

        (1)   Psychopathology, including: impaired reality testing, sociopathy, impaired interpersonal boundaries, personality disorder, substance abuse

        (2)   Immaturity, lack of commitment or dependability

e.   Family member(s) unprepared for roles, as evidenced by:

        (1)   Immaturity

        (2)   Inadequate educational, vocational, social development

        (3)   Lack of knowledge of role requirements and boundaries, parenting skills, interpersonal skills, or healthy behavior (response options)

        (4)   Impaired self-concept

        (5)   History as victim or passive participant in family violence

        (6)   Reared in family with dysfunctional communication patterns

f.   Family members with limited or absent opportunities to fulfill personal needs, as evidenced by:

        (1)   Pressure to meet others' needs to exclusion of personal needs

        (2)   Family member experiencing overwhelming personal needs, dependence

        (3)   Repeated pattern of violence because, although painful, the known represents security

        (4)   Role requiring actions interfering with meeting personal needs (e.g., mother home all day with small children, elderly parent; caretaker must work and child care inadequate; working more than one job and adopting submissive, passive attitude)

        (5)   Inadequate resources available to meet personal needs

2. Be alert for signs and symptoms of family violence, including:
    a. Evidence of physical injury:
        (1) Bruises, black eyes
        (2) Broken bones, frequent fractures
        (3) Burns, cuts
        (4) Skin breakdown in sedentary individuals
        (5) Limited range of motion, trouble ambulating and doing routine tasks
        (6) Complaints of pain, injury
    b. Evidence of abuse and neglect:
        (1) Untreated illness; absence of prophylactic care
        (2) Person, clothing, and environment of dependents not clean and maintained
        (3) Inadequate or inconsistent meeting of nutritional needs
        (4) Lack of supervision for family members
        (5) Reports of questionable events or practices from family or community members
        (6) Frequent absences from school or work with questionable or omitted explanations
        (7) Lack of social contacts, nonparticipation in activities
    c. Evidence of child sexual abuse:
        (1) Chronic genitourinary infections
        (2) Sexually transmitted disease symptoms
        (3) Irritated or swollen genitals
        (4) Irritated or swollen rectum (anal sex)
        (5) Sore throat, hyperactive gag reflex, vomiting (oral sex)
        (6) Weight gain or loss to affect attractiveness to abuser (by victim or observer)
    d. Characteristics associated with family violence:
        (1) Isolation, acute and chronic withdrawal (e.g., unwillingness to invite others to home, lack of friends or social outlets)
        2) Secretiveness, reluctance to talk about family and home life
        (3) Evidence of fear, intimidation, tension, and anxiety (e.g., jumpiness and nightmares)
        (4) Evidence of chronic anger, frustration, and displaced rage
        (5) Expressions of hopelessness, helplessness
        (6) Submissive, passive attitude
        (7) Failure to use problem-solving strategies
        (8) Lethargy and lack of motivation
        (9) Regression
3. Remain alert for evidence of sexually inappropriate behavior, overexcitement, and conflict, such as:

a. Reports of incest or rape
b. Sexual talk and behavior by young children
c. Discomfort with or avoidance of sexual contact
d. Impaired marital relationship and adult sexual relationships
e. Pornography, especially child pornography

4. Inquire about situations often associated with family violence; specific questions could include:
   a. Ask a child, "What happens to you when you do something wrong?"
   b. Ask a family member, "How do family disagreements affect you?"
5. Ensure privacy and confidentiality during questioning, and take a nonjudgmental, empathic approach to foster trust and openness.
6. Assess your own personal feelings and cognitive responses to family violence, which may involve:
   a. Reactivation of personal memories and issues around violence or abuse
   b. Negative affect: anger, blame, denial, being overwhelmed, avoidance, frustration, hopelessness, fear, disgust
   c. Positive affect: hope, support, caring, helpfulness, commitment, understanding
   d. Lack of confidence in professional ability to intervene

B. **Analysis and nursing diagnoses**
   1. Accurate analysis depends on knowledge of the phenomena of family violence, family dynamics, and application of the nursing process.
   2. Also important is knowledge of resources available to assist dysfunctional families.
   3. Pertinent North American Nursing Diagnosis Association (NANDA) nursing diagnoses could include:
      a. Nursing diagnoses made to promote safety and physical health:
         (1) High Risk for Violence
         (2) High Risk for Physical Injury
         (3) Health Management Deficit
         (4) Tissue Integrity: Impaired
         (5) High Risk for Infection
         (6) Altered Nutrition
         (7) Altered Comfort: Pain
         (8) Sleep Pattern Disturbance
         (9) Psychoactive Substance Use Disorder: Dependence
      b. Nursing diagnoses made to identify individuals' needs for intervention
         (1) Ineffective Individual Coping
         (2) Social Isolation
         (3) Impaired Social Interaction

        (4)   Diversional Activity Deficit
        (5)   Self-Esteem Disturbance
        (6)   Fear
        (7)   Anticipatory Anxiety
        (8)   Anxiety
        (9)   Situational Depression
        (10)   Rape Trauma Syndrome
        (11)   Rape Trauma Syndrome: Compound or Silent Reactions
        (12)   Sexual Dysfunction
        (13)   Impaired Thought Processes
        (14)   Hopelessness
        (15)   Powerlessness

    c.   Nursing diagnoses made to facilitate intervention with the family system
        (1)   Altered Family Processes
        (2)   Self-Concept Disturbance: Role Performance
        (3)   High Risk for Altered Parenting
        (4)   Altered Parenting
        (5)   Family Coping: High Risk for Growth
        (6)   Family Coping: Compromised
        (7)   Family Coping: Disabling

    d.   Other nursing diagnoses tailored to the individual's and family's needs
        (1)   Impaired Adjustment
        (2)   Knowledge Deficit
        (3)   Noncompliance

C. **Planning and implementation**
    1.   Provide first aid or medical treatment to the victim as needed.
    2.   Collect assessment data and specimens for police when rape or other sexual abuse is suspected.
    3.   Provide reports to state protective services for child and elder abuse as required by law.
    4.   Select an intervention sequence based on immediacy of danger to the victim to ensure safety:
        a.   If violence or abuse is imminent, separate victim from aggressor:
           (1)   Emergency shelters, hospitals, and foster homes may be used.
           (2)   Removal of both victim and abuser from home minimizes victim's guilt and sense of responsibility.
        b.   Provide treatment before victim is returned to family environment.
        c.   If sufficient controls exist to prevent violence, victim may remain in home.

(1) When family violence is revealed, family may become more amenable to therapeutic influence, support, and change.

(2) Victim is not left alone with abuser.

5. Work to help resolve family dysfunction using various theoretic models as appropriate:
   a. Psychodynamic theories
      (1) Psychoanalytically oriented therapy
      (2) Transactional analysis
      (3) Gestalt therapy
   b. Family therapy
      (1) Bowen theory
      (2) Structural analysis
      (3) Minuchin theory
   c. Communication or interpersonal theories
   d. Educational frameworks
      (1) Parent education
      (2) Self-help models
   e. Individual and group contexts to facilitate learning and change
      (1) Family sessions, including marital therapy
      (2) Individual sessions for psychotherapy, counseling, play therapy, and art therapy
      (3) Group therapy for victims and offenders
      (4) Support groups that help members learn and monitor coping strategies (e.g., Parents Anonymous, Alcoholics Anonymous, Narcotics Anonymous, Parents Without Partners, and groups based on diagnosis [manic-depression, schizophrenia])

6. Provide individual therapy for victims that promotes coping with trauma and prevents future psychologic conflict:
   a. Promote ventilation and catharsis.
   b. Assist integration of experience of abuse and reestablishment of healthy self-concept.
   c. Assist moving from victim role to posture as functioning survivor.
   d. Assist survivor to understand his participation in abuse, if any:
      (1) Submissiveness, passivity
      (2) Provocation or encouragement
   e. Assist understanding of abuser's dynamics.
   f. Assist understanding of family patterns and dynamics that permit or promote violence or abuse.
   g. Assist development of self-protective abilities and other problem-solving strategies.

    h.   Provide support to victim for not tolerating abuse and taking steps toward growth.

    i.   Provide support and assistance in coping with contact with legal system; avoid revictimization.

    j.   When survivor is a child, intervene also with custodial parent(s):

        (1)   Information is provided about normal development.

        (2)   Information is provided about effective parenting.

    k.   When survivor is a child, provide nonverbal modalities:

        (1)   Play therapy; puppets or dolls

        (2)   Art therapy

    l.   Help children to deal with guilt and other effects of trauma.

        (1)   Child may develop conduct disorders as well as affective symptoms.

        (2)   Stress symptoms are identified as time-limited and part of the healing process.

        (3)   Child may regress.

        (4)   Child may develop negative attitude toward gender of abuser.

7.   Provide individual therapy for abusers that focuses on preventing violent behavior and repairing relationships.

    a.   Focus on accepting responsibility for behavior and maximizing efforts at change.

    b.   Provide support and assistance in coping with legal ramifications.

    c.   Provide information about healthy functioning:

        (1)   Problem-solving and coping strategies

        (2)   Effective parenting

        (3)   Interpersonal relationships and communication

        (4)   Individual needs

    d.   Assist to attain and maintain impulse control.

    e.   Support nonviolent attempts to interact with others and meet personal needs.

    f.   Provide treatment for personal psychopathology:

        (1)   Compliance taking antipsychotic medication or other psychotropics

        (2)   Substance abuse treatment

8.   Provide family therapy to involve observers and to address system issues.

    a.   Identify dysfunctional communication styles.

    b.   Discover intergenerational patterns.

    c.   Explore relationships.

    d.   Explore healthy alternative behaviors.

    e.   Support healthy aspects of family interaction.

       f.   Realign relationships.
       g.   Reduce stigmatizing role pressure.
       h.   Provide observers of violence support for their trauma.

9. Make appropriate referrals to treaters or agencies for intervention not personally conducted.
    a.   Assist family to identify and access community and personal resources:
       (1)   Community mental health centers
       (2)   Respite care services
    b.   Act as liaison for family and resources.
    c.   Coordinate efforts of various treaters.
    d.   Monitor effectiveness of intervention.

10. Act as responsible professional member of community by promoting social change.
    a.   Work to alleviate violence-promoting conditions:
       (1)   Poverty
       (2)   Inadequate housing, homelessness
       (3)   Underemployment
       (4)   Dysfunctional social attitudes
       (5)   Substance abuse
    b.   Work to develop and maintain resources for families so violence is prevented:
       (1)   Community mental health services, follow-up
       (2)   Respite care for elderly, mentally ill
       (3)   Child care services
       (4)   Foster care services
       (5)   Preventive education for children on appropriate interactions, avoiding abuse
       (6)   Volunteers, homemaker services
       (7)   Support groups
    c.   Support and promote legal and legislative systems efforts to eliminate family violence.

D. **Evaluation**
1. Precipitating factors for violence or abuse are reduced or eliminated.
2. Improvement in family system interaction is evidenced.
3. Abusive or violent behavior is reduced or eliminated.

Bibliography

Janosik, E. H., & Davies, E. L. (1987). *Psychiatric mental health nursing.* Boston: Jones & Bartlett.

Johnson, B. S. (1989). *Psychiatric-mental health nursing: Adaptation and growth* (2nd ed.). Philadelphia: J. B. Lippincott.

Stuart, G. W., & Sundeen, S. J. (1987). *Principles and practice of psychiatric nursing* (3rd ed.). St. Louis: C. V. Mosby.

Wilson, H. S., & Kneisl, C. R. (1988). *Psychiatric nursing* (3rd ed.). Menlo Park, CA: Addison-Wesley.

STUDY QUESTIONS

1. The Smith family recently moved to town. Susie, at age 11 the youngest, has fresh bruises every week. When the parents were asked about her black eye, Mrs. Smith interrupted her husband to say that Susie is a clumsy, daydreaming, accident-prone child. Her two older brothers don't seem to notice the bruises. They replied with, "I dunno" and "She's always doing something stupid" when peers asked about the new black eye. Susie was sent to the school nurse when she complained of dizziness and nausea before lunch. A school nurse first seeing Susie walk into the office would appropriately could recognize feeling
   a. concerned
   b. anger, because the nurse was about to go to lunch
   c. critical of her having a black eye
   d. all of the above

2. Aware of Susie's reputation as clumsy, the school nurse should take which of the following appropriate actions?
   a. Notify playground monitors to watch out for Susie.
   b. Teach Susie about being careful and thinking before acting.
   c. Be alert to the possibility of child abuse and gather more data.
   d. Consult with Susie's teacher about creating a safe environment.

3. The nurse's priority focus in assessing Susie's situation would be to determine
   a. how quickly Susie's mother can arrive to take her home
   b. whether the black eye is self-inflicted or caused by an accident or assault
   c. whether Susie will be able to concentrate on schoolwork after resting
   d. if signs of concussion (due to trauma) requiring further treatment are present

4. When asked where her black eye came from, Susie replies, "I was a bad girl and made Daddy mad." The nurse should consider this information with which of the following correlates of family violence?
   a. female child, history of bruises, recent move
   b. female child, high socioeconomic status (SES) neighborhood, recent move
   c. disobedience, low SES neighborhood, two brothers
   d. childhood lying, high SES neighborhood, rumored clumsiness

5. Susie's mother tells the nurse that Mr. Smith hit Susie when he had been drinking, and that she has almost talked him into contacting AA. She asks the nurse not to interfere so Mr. Smith does not get angry and refuse alcohol treatment. Which of the following would be the nurse's best response?
   a. promising not to intervene if Mr. Smith attends AA that night
   b. commending Mrs. Smith's efforts and promising to let her handle the situation
   c. commending Mrs. Smith's efforts and planning to contact protective services through established channels
   d. confronting Mrs. Smith's failure to protect her daughter and planning to contact protective services through established channels

6. The mother reports that Mr. Smith "disciplined" Susie for not getting him breakfast, stating that Susie "should have known" to do so on Saturday despite being told on Thursday never to prepare him food. Which of the following would be an appropriate response from the nurse?
   a. Acknowledge that children should meet their parents' needs.
   b. Teach Mrs. Smith that children need consistent limits and structure.
   c. Admit that Susie deserved to be hit

but state that Mr. Smith went overboard by giving her a black eye.

   d. Teach Mrs. Smith that corporal punishment is appropriately administered to the buttocks, not the face.

7. Mary takes excellent care of her mother, who is bedridden. She voluntarily quit her part-time job and spends all her time at home to be with her. Both mother and daughter interact only with other family members. Mary reports to the nurse that her mother "can be difficult" and refuses to cooperate with activities of daily living. In fact, during a bed bath, her mother slapped Mary. Mary felt guilty about her impulse to slap her mother back. She commented, "You must think I'm awful. But then, I'm probably making a big deal out of nothing." Mary's willingness to discuss the episode may stem from

   a. her discomfort with her response to her mother

   b. her need to ventilate frustration and helplessness

   c. her trust in the nurse

   d. all of the above

8. The nurse's best first response to Mary would be

   a. "Yes. After all, you didn't actually hit her."

   b. "You have a difficult situation on your hands."

   c. "You'd better not start slapping your mother."

   d. "Have you thought about nursing home placement?"

9. Mary's mother likely would best benefit from

   a. discussing her reasons for not cooperating

   b. having more time alone to consider the effects of her behavior

   c. being told that she could be charged with assault

   d. being approached as if she were a recalcitrant child

10. Which of the following would impair the mother's ability to participate in problem solving?

   a. organic mental disorder associated with aging

   b. the desire to have suggestions written down

   c. extreme old age

   d. insisting the nurse visit after a favorite television program is over

11. Carol, aged 17, has been having trouble since she started 7th grade—skipping class, acting sullen with adults (especially male teachers). She is only eating one meal a day and is sleeping poorly. Her mother entered the hospital for surgery on Monday, and Carol ran away to a friend's house after school, where she acted frightened of her friend's older brothers. Carol then asked her neighbor, a nurse, if she could stay with her, and then blurted out, "I can't be home when Mom's not there. Uncle Bill bothers me and won't stay in his own room." Based on this information, the nurse should strongly suspect which of the following ?

   a. She is bothered by her Uncle's teasing.

   b. She prefers to have the house to herself.

   c. She is psychotic.

   d. She may be an incest victim.

12. Assuming that Carol has been sexually abused, what would most likely be the significance of her change in eating habits?

   a. It is due to worry over her mother's illness.

   b. It is not significant clinical data.

   c. It is an attempt to make herself less attractive by losing weight.

   d. It is of no significance unless she loses more than 5% of her body weight.

ANSWER KEY

1. **Correct response: d**
   The nurse should acknowledge all personal responses to this patient and her situation, not just caring responses.
   a, b, and c. All of these responses should be acknowledged.
   Application/Health promotion/Assessment

2. **Correct response: c**
   The professional nurse is aware of the issue of family violence, collects sufficient information to make nursing diagnoses and personally makes a professional analysis of information obtained.
   a, b, and d. The other interventions would be premature, based on limited and unsubstantiated data.
   Knowledge/Safe care/Assessment

3. **Correct response: d**
   The priority is to ensure physiologic health, through referral for medical treatment if indicated. Psychosocial assessment is done when physical well-being is addressed.
   Application/Physiologic/Assessment

4. **Correct response: a**
   Female children are more often abused than male children. Victims of family abuse commonly have a history of injuries. A recent move could indicate family stress and social isolation.
   b, c, and d. Although family violence can be associated with financial stress, it also occurs in families with high incomes. The child relates her father to the injury, not her brothers; brother–sister abuse is less common. The nurse has not observed the girl being clumsy; this is the mother's report and may indicate denial. Children's reports of abuse must be investigated and

disproved, not automatically rejected as lying.
   Knowledge/Psychosocial/Analysis (Dx)

5. **Correct response: c**
   Nurses belong to the group of professionals required by law to report child abuse.
   a and b. The nurse is obligated by law to report all cases of child abuse.
   d. Supporting family members' efforts at problem solving yields better therapeutic effect than does a blaming or accusing response.
   Comprehension/Safe care/Implementation

6. **Correct response: b**
   Providing information on effective parenting behavior promotes psychologic security and safety for the child and improves parents' coping skills.
   a. This response would promote role blurring and perpetuate dysfunctional expectations.
   c and d. These responses indicate approval of corporal punishment, which communicates that it is all right to hit someone to get what you want.
   Application/Psychosocial/Implementation

7. **Correct response: d**
   All of these factors influence Mary's ability to make herself available for intervention.
   a, b, and c. All of these factors are significant.
   Analysis/Psychosocial/Analysis (Dx)

8. **Correct response: b**
   This response offers empathic support, which encourages further discussion.
   a. This response minimizes Mary's concerns and discourages problem solving.
   c. This response is critical and would interfere with developing an alliance, and it also reflects doubt

about Mary's continued coping abilities.

d. This response also de-skills Mary and would represent a premature intervention at this point.

Analysis/Psychosocial/Implementation

9. **Correct response: a**
   This approach would provide assessment data and involve the mother in developing solutions to the problem identified.

   b. This approach incorrectly recommends further isolation for someone with already limited contacts.
   c. This approach is threatening and could escalate a power struggle.
   d. Interacting with elderly people as if they are children is a devaluing abuse in itself.

Analysis/Psychosocial/Planning

10. **Correct response: a**
    Many elderly victims or potential victims are psychologically impaired.

    b and d. These offer ways to incorporate the mother's needs into the planning, and so are incorrect.
    c. Old age in itself does not prevent problem solving.

Knowledge/Physiologic/Implementation

11. **Correct response: d**
    The evidence in this situation points to a possible incestuous situation.

    a. Carol's statement that Uncle Bill "doesn't stay in his room" points to a deeper problem than teasing.
    b. Carol's statement mentions Uncle Bill specifically as bothering her, suggesting that there is more involved than wanting to be alone.
    c. Although data suggesting conduct disorder are provided, there is no reason to consider Carol as psychotic.

Comprehension/Health promotion/Analysis (Dx)

12. **Correct response: c**
    Weight change (either loss or gain) is associated with body image and is a commonly seen response in incest victims.

    a. According to the information presented, Carol's change in eating habits began before her mother's hospitalization.
    b and d. Any unhealthy eating habit should be addressed as soon as it becomes apparent.

Application/Physiologic/Analysis (Dx)

Childhood and Adolescent Disorders

I.   Overview

A.   Definitions

   1.   Childhood: a period usually defined as beginning during the preschool years (age 3 or 4 years) and extending through the elementary and middle school years (around age 12 years)

   2.   Adolescence: a period usually defined as beginning at 12 or 13 years of age and extending through the teenage years, even to 20 or 21 years of age

B.   Basic concepts: Developmental theory (Erikson)

   1.   Trust vs. mistrust

      a.   Age : birth to age 1½ years

       b.   Task: to learn to trust the world to care for him or her in a consistent and predictable manner

       c.   Develops confidence in the world, which adds to his or her sense of self

       d.   Develops from the mother–child relationship

  2.   Autonomy vs. shame and doubt

       a.   Age: 1½ to 3 years

       b.   Task: to develop a sense of independence and self-control without a loss of self-esteem

       c.   Autonomy: characterized by self-expression and cooperation

       d.   When overcontrolled, the child experiences shame and doubt, which are characterized by rage, stubbornness, fears, obsessive-compulsive behavior.

  3.   Initiative vs. guilt

       a.   Age: 3 to 5 years

       b.   Task: to be active for the sake of being on the go; to test what may be done

  4.   Industry vs. inferiority and inadequacy

       a.   Age: 6 to 12 years

       b.   Task: to learn to be productive, to work, to compete

  5.   Identity vs. role confusion

       a.   Age: 12 to 20 years

       b.   Task: to develop personal, sexual, and occupational identity

C. **Basic concepts: Family psychodynamics**

  1.   Severe emotional problems in children and teens are thought to involve family system elements (i.e., the patient is a symptom bearer).

  2.   Several family system factors are commonly seen, including:

       a.   Overanxious or rigid parenting

       b.   Conflictual relationships

       c.   Double-bind or inconsistent communication patterns

       d.   Blurring of ego boundaries or enmeshed relationships; poor differentiation of individual member identity

D. **Factors associated with childhood and adolescent disorders**

  1.   Biologic factors in children include:

       a.   Congenital disorders leading to mental retardation or hyperactivity

       b.   Substance abuse results (e.g., cocaine-addicted infants or fetal alcohol syndrome)

  2.   Biologic factors in adolescence include:

       a.   Hormonal changes affecting growth (body image), mood, and drives

       b.   Dramatic change in genital development (psychosexuality and body image)

    3. Sociocultural factors in children include:
        a. Family system issues (see Section I.C)
        b. Acceptance and achievement in school, which may affect ego development
        c. Environmental factors (poverty, neglect, inadequate basic needs) that can negatively affect healthy development
    4. Sociocultural factors in adolescence include:
        a. Family system issues (see Section I.C)
        b. Development of own identity and separation from family
        c. Acceptance by peers, which plays a critical role in behavior and may lead to rebellious or illegal activities
        d. Environmental factors (e.g., poverty, lack of guidelines, inadequate basic needs) that may lead to rebellious or illegal activities

E. General characteristics of childhood and adolescent disorders
    1. Impaired growth and development patterns
    2. Physical illness
    3. Lack of or unusual relatedness with peers or significant others
    4. Overachievement or underachievement
    5. Overinvolvement or underinvolvement with age-related activities
    6. Family system problems or conflicts
    7. Expressions of self-disgust, sadness
    8. Impaired age-appropriate reality testing
    9. Poor impulse control
    10. Sexual acting-out
    11. Aggressive and destructive behavior

II. Types of childhood and adolescent disorders
  A. Developmental disorders
    1. Mental retardation
        a. Subaverage intelligence (IQ of 70 or less)
        b. Impaired social and communication skills and an inability to be self-sufficient
        c. Onset before one's 18th birthday
    2. Pervasive developmental disorders: autistic disorders
        a. Impairment in interpersonal relationships; strong desire to be alone
        b. Language used in an idiosyncratic manner; unconventional meaning of words, continuous repetition of words (echolalia), and use of "I" for "you" and vice-versa (pronoun reversal)
        c. Like things to stay the same, can't tolerate change
        d. Interest: narrow and unimaginative
        e. Body movements: repetitive and restricted
        f. Onset in the first 30 months of life
    3. Special developmental disorders

      a. Developmental disorders in the areas of academia, language, and speech as well as in motor skills

      b. Not attributable to mental retardation, pervasive developmental disorders, or educational deficiencies

B. Emotional disorders

  1. Depression

      a. Prolonged sadness, apathy, crying

      b. Anhedonia

      c. Low self-esteem

      d. Social isolation

      e. Poor concentration, reduced attention span

      f. Suicidal ideation

      g. Somatic complaints

      h. Irritability

      i. Acting-out behavior

      j. Reduced performance in school

  2. Suicidal behavior

      a. Youth suicide increasing

      b. Second leading cause of death in the 15- to 24-year-old age group

      c. Warning signs: depression and hopelessness; losses of significant others; stressful family environment

  3. Anxiety disorders

      a. Separation anxiety disorders: characterized by excessive anxiety and worry related to separation; refusal to go to school and to be alone; duration of at least 2 weeks; onset before the 18th birthday

      b. Avoidant disorder of childhood or adolescence: characterized by extreme shyness around strangers, which impairs social interactions, although there is desire for social contacts; onset at the beginning of school

  4. Schizophrenia

      a. In childhood, symptoms are similar to those found in adults, except hallucinations and delusions are rare

      b. In adolescents, symptoms are similar to those found in adults

  5. Substance abuse disorder

      a. Deterioration in social and academic functioning

      b. Changes in usual manner of behaving: bizarre behavior, aggressive behavior, extremely sedated behavior

C. Disruptive behavioral disorders

  1. Attention deficit–hyperactivity disorders

      a. Restlessness, short attention span, easily distracted, impulsiveness, hyperactivity, poor concentration, failure to complete tasks, inability to wait

        b.   Duration of at least 6 months

        c.   Onset before 7th birthday

    2.   Conduct disorders

        a.   Disregard for the rights of others and for rules, physical aggressiveness, absence of guilt, irritability, low tolerance for frustration, low self-esteem, fire setting, stealing, running away, lying, sexually acting-out, trouble with the law

        b.   Duration of at least 6 months

        c.   Onset before 18th birthday

    3.   Oppositional defiant disorders

        a.   Argumentative, swearing, resentful and angry, low tolerance level, defiant, hostile

        b.   Duration of at least 6 months

        c.   Onset before 18th birthday

D.   **Eating disorders**

    1.   Anorexia nervosa

        a.   Distorted body image: views self as fat, preoccupied with weight

        b.   Fears gaining weight so reduces food intake; refuses to eat the elaborate meals he or she prepares

        c.   Refusal to maintain a normal body weight

        d.   No loss of appetite

        e.   Medical complications (hypotension, hypothermia, metabolic changes, death)

        f.   Amenorrhea

        g.   Use of laxatives, self-induced vomiting

        h.   Onset in adolescence

        i.   More common in girls than boys

    2.   Bulimia nervosa

        a.   Repeated episodes of binge eating (at least two binge-eating episodes per week for 3 months)

        b.   No control of overeating

        c.   Self-induced vomiting, use of laxatives and strict diets

        d.   Persistent concern about weight

III. **Nursing process in childhood and adolescent disorders**

   A.   Assessment

    1.   Note abnormal physiologic responses, such as:

        a.   Somatic complaints

        b.   Decreased eating, binging or vomiting, weight loss

        c.   Substance abuse symptoms

    2.   Explore for behavioral responses, such as:

        a.   Discipline or conduct problems

        b.   Sexual acting-out

        c.   Withdrawal or social isolation

        d.   Aggressive, destructive behavior

        e.   Poor or unusually strong relatedness with peers/significant others

        f.   Academic problems or truancy

        g.   Poor impulse control, rebellion and defiance

        h.   Substance use or abuse

   3.   Note abnormal cognitive responses, such as:

        a.   Lack of reality testing

        b.   Poor attention span, learning problems

        c.   Language and speech difficulties

        d.   Unusual thought processes, suspicion

   4.   Observe for such affective responses as:

        a.   Mood swings: elation to sadness, depression

        b.   Intense emotions: rage, sadness

        c.   Feelings of hopelessness; suicidal thoughts and feelings

        d.   Lack of affect

B. **Analysis and nursing diagnoses**

   1.   Accurate analysis depends on a knowledge of growth and development.

   2.   It also requires consideration of the child's or adolescent's age and emotional maturity, as well as the family's perceptions and responses to symptoms.

   3.   Pertinent North American Nursing Diagnosis Association (NANDA) diagnoses may include:

        a.   Ineffective Individual Coping

           (1)   Related to being easily distractible

           (2)   Related to having a short attention span

        b.   Altered Nutrition: Less Than Body Requirements

           (1)   Related to decreased desire to eat

           (2)   Related to induced vomiting

        c.   Social Isolation

           (1)   Related to inadequate social skills

           (2)   Related to feelings of inadequacy or inferiority

        d.   High Risk for Violence: Self-Directed

           (1)   Related to self-disgust

           (2)   Related to feeling of hopelessness

        e.   Impaired Social Interaction

           (1)   Related to inability to follow rules

           (2)   Related to testing the limits

        f.   High Risk for Violence: Directed at Others

           (1)   Related to hitting others

           (2)   Related to feelings of anger and frustration

C. **Planning and implementation**

   1.   Always involve parents in treatment plan to increase the likelihood of parental support.

   2.   Provide psychoeducation, covering information about normal development and the current knowledge regarding the disorder, its treatment, and its management at home.

3. Alleviate feelings of guilt and self-blame.
4. Encourage expression of helplessness, confusion, and other feelings and concerns.
5. Inform both the parents and the child or adolescent of what information will be shared with the parents.
6. Listen empathically; be supportive.
7. Do not take the side of either the parent or the child or adolescent.
8. Do not assume the parental role.
9. As appropriate, involve siblings in psychoeducation and expression of feelings and concerns.
10. Support strengths of family members.
11. Promote clear, honest, straightforward communication; use simple terminology to explain complex concepts.
12. Avoid power struggles by calmly stating expectations and consequences.
13. Establish contracts with adolescents to promote sense of control and autonomy.
14. Be aware of transference and countertransference issues:
    a. Transference: an unconscious response in which the patient experiences feelings toward the nurse originally associated with a significant other
    b. Countertransference: an emotional reaction in the nurse toward the patient that is inappropriate to the therapeutic relationship
15. Recognize feelings (anger, sadness, frustration) and deal with them constructively.
16. Use silence constructively; keep in mind that prolonged silence can increase tension.
17. Focus inpatient treatment on the setting:
    a. Milieu therapy: construct a safe, structured environment with daily schedules and behavior modification.
    b. Behavior modification: positively reinforce acceptable behavior with tangible and social rewards.
18. Recognize the social stigma associated with psychiatric hospitalization and psychotherapy, and assist the patient to verbalize his reaction to the psychiatric hospitalization and stigma.
19. Use the cognitive model to explain the relationship between thoughts, feelings, and behavior (i.e., thoughts lead to feelings and behavior, but a person does not have to act on feelings or thoughts).
20. Provide play therapy for children:
    a. Provide a safe environment for the exploration and working-through of conflicts and feelings.

    b.   Use toys, paper, crayons, and other items as the medium of expression; minimize talking.

    c.   Permit the child to set the pace.

    d.   Be facilitative and supportive.

  21. Make appropriate referrals, which may include:

    a.   Psychologic assessment

    b.   Group psychotherapy

    c.   Parental support group

    d.   Family therapy

    e.   Community resource agencies

    f.   Big Brother or Big Sister Organizations

D. **Evaluation**

  1. The patient and family exhibit improved coping skills.

  2. The patient demonstrates adequate nutritional intake.

  3. The patient reports and exhibits improved social interaction patterns.

  4. The patient verbalizes and exhibits decreased propensity for self-harm and violence toward others.

Bibliography

Janosik, E. H., & Davies, E. L. (1987). *Psychiatric mental health nursing.* Boston: Jones & Bartlett.

Johnson, B. S. (1989). *Psychiatric-mental health nursing: Adaptation and growth* (2nd ed.). Philadelphia: J. B. Lippincott.

Stuart, G. W., & Sundeen, S. J. (1987). *Principles and practice of psychiatric nursing* (3rd ed.). St. Louis: C. V. Mosby.

Wilson, H. S., & Kneisl, C. R. (1988). *Psychiatric nursing* (3rd ed.). Menlo Park, CA: Addison-Wesley.

STUDY QUESTIONS

1. Jane, aged 9, was brought to the hospital after attempting to hang herself in her parents' basement. The nurse's first intervention should be to
   a. Talk to her parents alone to alleviate their fears.
   b. Talk to Jane alone to provide immediate relief of her pain.
   c. Talk to both Jane and her parents together for a brief period before spending time with Jane alone.
   d. Talk to her teacher to obtain her academic records.

2. The next day, the nurse decides to bring in several toys, including a doll house, a mother doll, a father doll, and a child doll, as well as papers and pencils. The nurse's decision is based on the assumption that children
   a. communicate better verbally
   b. express their conflict nonverbally through their play
   c. need to be preoccupied with things
   d. have more fun when they are playing

3. Jane rearranges some of the furniture in the doll house and places the child doll in a room by itself. The nurse's initial response is to
   a. Say, "No! Place the doll with her parents."
   b. Say nothing, just observe Jane's play.
   c. Ask, "Why is the child doll by herself?"
   d. Say, "Let me read you a story."

4. Prolonged silence during the initial stage of the nurse–child relationship is
   a. therapeutic because it indicates interest
   b. therapeutic because it respects the child's autonomy
   c. nontherapeutic because it allows the child to progress at her own pace
   d. nontherapeutic because it enhances the child's anxiety

5. Scott, aged 13, frequently fights with other children, lies, steals, and breaks rules. Which of the following medical and nursing diagnoses most likely would be appropriate for Scott?
   a. High Risk for Conduct Disorder and Violence: Directed at Others
   b. Conduct disorder and Social Isolation
   c. Depression and Social Isolation
   d. Disturbance in Depression and Self-Concept: Body Image

6. Even though Scott is chronologically in Erikson's Identity vs. Role Confusion stage, his behavior is most typical of
   a. Trust vs. Mistrust
   b. Initiative vs. Guilt
   c. Autonomy vs. Shame and Doubt
   d. Industry vs. Inferiority

7. The nursing process includes this plan: Scott will eat all meals in his room. Which of the following statements best describes this plan?
   a. It doesn't address Scott's defiant acting-out behavior.
   b. It addresses Scott's problem by providing time out from an overstimulating environment.
   c. It addresses Scott's problem by allowing for development of self-control.
   d. It doesn't address Scott's problem of social isolation.

8. The nurse's most appropriate initial intervention for Scott's fighting would be to
   a. Talk to Scott each time he hits another child.
   b. Anticipate and neutralize all potentially explosive situations.
   c. Take away his privileges.
   d. Ignore small infractions of the rules.

9. The nurse knows this intervention is successful if Scott
   a. eats his meals
   b. talks to peers
   c. sits alone watching television
   d. plays cooperatively without fighting

10. John, aged 7, has a diagnosis of attention deficit–hyperactivity disorder. He is most likely to exhibit which of the following symptoms?
    a. restlessness, decreased attention span, and distractibility
    b. hyperactivity, failure to complete tasks, and physical aggressiveness
    c. impulsiveness, anhedonia, and shyness
    d. poor concentration, decreased attention span, and somatic complaints

11. After obtaining information about John's symptoms and observing his interactions with people and objects, the nurse says to John's parents, "Often parents try many things to help their child before bringing him to the hospital. What things have you tried?" This intervention is
    a. not therapeutic because it will not provide useful assessment data
    b. not therapeutic because the parents are not in treatment
    c. therapeutic because it reduces the overwhelming tension the nurse is experiencing
    d. therapeutic because it provides information about the impact of the symptoms on the family

12. John's parents say they have tried everything, and nothing seems to work. They add that they are more irritable and are blaming each other for John's behavior. Which of the following actions would be most appropriate for the nurse to take at this time?
    a. Listen to their concerns but quickly disengage.
    b. Encourage them to talk to John's physician.
    c. Refer them for psychoeducation.
    d. Tell them that they are overreacting.

13. The treatment team's recommendations for John's parents likely would include which of the following?
    a. Give John clear and simple directions.
    b. Talk to John for at least 1 hour each day.
    c. Encourage more peer interaction for John.
    d. Encourage them to plan more family activities.

14. A safe, structured environment that provides daily schedules and promotes growth and development through constant and consistent feedback describes
    a. supportive therapy
    b. milieu therapy
    c. psychoanalytic therapy
    d. dynamic therapy

ANSWER KEY

1. **Correct response: c**
   This allows the nurse to observe the family as a unit and to obtain some general information before spending time with Jane alone.
   a and b. The nurse needs to establish herself or himself as a neutral intervener who is interested in the family as an adaptive functioning unit.
   d. Even though Jane's academic records will be useful at a later point in assessment, they are not of primary concern initially.
   Application/Psychosocial/Implementation

2. **Correct response: b**
   Play therapy provides a medium for the child to nonverbally explore and develop strategies for dealing with conflict.
   a. Children often have problems verbalizing their pain.
   c and d. The purpose of play therapy is to enhance healthy development, not to keep the child busy or provide entertainment.
   Application/Psychosocial/Implementation

3. **Correct response: b**
   The nurse communicates acceptance and a desire to understand by allowing the child to set the pace during play therapy. In addition, nurses need to observe for patterns in the child's play.
   a, c, and d. These actions would not permit the child to establish the pace.
   Application/Psychosocial/Implementation

4. **Correct response: d**
   Silence during the initial stage of the nurse–child relationship inadvertently enhances the child's anxiety.
   a and b. Prolonged silence doesn't communicate interest or respect a child's autonomy.
   c. Prolonged silence hinders the child's progress.
   Analysis/Psychosocial/Implementation

5. **Correct response: a**
   The symptoms described are typically found in children with conduct disorder and the potential for violent behavior.
   b, c, and d. Social isolation, depression, and altered body image are not typically characteristic of conduct disorder. However, children and adolescents who are depressed may exhibit conduct disorder in addition to sadness and hopelessness.
   Comprehension/Psychosocial/Analysis (Dx)

6. **Correct response: c**
   Defiance is more characteristic of the Autonomy vs. Shame and Doubt stage than of the stages mentioned in responses a, b, and d.
   a, b, and d. Defiance is not characteristic of these stages.
   Comprehension/Psychosocial/Analysis (Dx)

7. **Correct response: a**
   This plan of having Scott eat in his room doesn't lead to interventions that would assist Scott to learn more effective coping strategies.
   b and c. Neither of these actions would contribute to Scott's repertoire of adaptive behaviors.
   d. This action would be inappropriate because Scott is not socially withdrawn.
   Analysis/Psychosocial/Planning

8. **Correct response: b**
   The nurse's responsibility is to create a safe environment by anticipating and neutralizing extraneous stressors.
   a and d. These actions would only reinforce Scott's fighting behavior.
   c. This action would not provide alternative behavior for Scott to practice.
   Application/Safe care/Implementation

9. **Correct response: d**
   Scott's cooperative, nonviolent behav-

ior would be indicative of adaptive behavior.

 a, b, and c. These criteria do not evaluate Scott's fighting behavior.

Application/Safe care/Evaluation

10. *Correct response: a*
Attention deficit–hyperactivity disorder is characterized by all of these symptoms.

 b, c, and d. Physical aggressiveness, anhedonia, shyness, and somatic complaints are not associated with attention deficit–hyperactivity disorders.

Knowledge/Psychosocial/Assessment

11. *Correct response: d*
It is important to obtain assessment data on the family's perceptions and reactions to the child's symptoms. These data will assist the nurse in developing an individualized treatment plan for the child.

 a, b, and c. These descriptions are not applicable to this approach.

Analysis/Psychosocial/Assessment

12. *Correct response: c*
Psychoeducation provides the family with useful information about the child's disorder and what the family can do to manage the child at home. It also addresses typical parental responses to the child's disorder, which helps to alleviate guilt and blaming.

 a, b, and d. These actions would communicate disinterest and could exacerbate the parents' confusion and sense of helplessness.

Application/Psychosocial/Implementation

13. *Correct response: a*
Children who are hyperactive need simple, concrete directions to help them focus their attention.

 b. Short interactions generally are more effective than prolonged ones.

 c and d. Social isolation is not John's problem.

Analysis/Psychosocial/Implementation

14. *Correct response: b*
Milieu therapy creates a structured environment that promotes growth.

 a, c, and d. The focus of these therapeutic approaches is not on a therapeutic community but rather on a one-to-one therapeutic relationship.

Comprehension/Safe care/Implementation

Organic Mental Disorders

11

I. Overview

A. Definitions

1. Organic mental disorder: mental or emotional condition that is physiologic in nature and results in potentially permanent tissue damage; sometimes referred to as brain syndrome

2. Organic mental syndrome: mental or emotional condition of no specific, known etiology

3. Functional disorder: mental or emotional condition thought to be psychosocial in nature

4. Cognition: the ability to think and reason, the distinguishing feature of human beings in the animal phylum

5. Orientation: the ability to relate self to the sphere of time, place, and person

6. Confusion: a condition characterized by disorientation, memory deficits, poor reality testing, and inappropriate verbal statements

B. Basic concepts

1. Delirium is an acute brain syndrome that has a rapid onset; with prompt treatment, it is usually reversible.
2. Dementia is a chronic brain syndrome that has a gradual onset and is usually progressive, causing irreversible tissue damage.
3. Delirium may occur at any age; dementia is most common in persons over age 65.
4. Delirium may occur in those persons already suffering from dementia and may become a dementia if untreated.
5. Depression may mimic symptoms of delirium and dementia.
6. General characteristics of organic mental disorders include:
   a. Deficits in orientation
   b. Deficits in memory
   c. Deficits in intellectual function: problem solving, reasoning
   d. Deficits in judgment
   e. Deficits in affect

C. Etiology

1. Factors associated with delirium may include:
   a. Hypoxias resulting from anemia; occult bleeding; deficiencies of iron, folic acid, or vitamin B_{12}; dehydration; hyperthermia or hypothermia; lung pathology; hypotension or hypertension; or increased intracranial pressure
   b. Metabolic disorders resulting from hormonal imbalance, endocrine dysfunction (thyroid, pancreas, adrenal), or nutritional factors
   c. Toxins and infections resulting from kidney pathology, hepatic pathology, drug interactions, alcoholism, or viral or bacteriologic stressors
   d. Structural changes resulting from tumors, trauma, surgery, or childbirth
   e. Environmental factors resulting from sensory overload or deprivation, sensory changes caused by poor eyesight and hearing, or isolation
2. Factors associated with dementias may include:
   a. All of the above stressors for delirium, if untreated or untreatable
   b. Vascular diseases such as arteriosclerosis, atherosclerosis, and cerebrovascular accidents
   c. Neurologic diseases such as Huntington's chorea, Parkinson's disease, neurosyphilis, Pick's disease, multi-infarct dementia, Alzheimer's disease, and cerebral atrophy

II. Types of organic mental disorders or syndromes

A. Delirium
1. Impaired consciousness and cognition; reduced ability to maintain attention
2. Hallucinations, illusions
3. Incoherence
4. Agitation or somnolence
5. Disorientation and confusion

B. Dementia (also primary degenerative, Alzheimer's type; multi-infarct dementia)
1. Loss of intellectual abilities interfering with functional ability
2. Impaired memory and orientation
3. Difficulties with reasoning and judgment
4. Personality change

C. Amnestic syndrome
1. Impaired short- and long-term memory
2. Absence of clouded consciousness or impaired intellectual ability

D. Organic delusional disorder
1. Presence of delusions in normal state of consciousness
2. Absence of deterioration of intellectual functioning

E. Organic hallucinosis
1. Persistent hallucinations in normal state of consciousness
2. Absence of deteriorated intellectual functioning, mood disorder, or delusions

F. Organic affective (mood) disorder
1. Disturbance in mood: either manic or depressive
2. Absence of impaired intellectual ability, hallucinations, or delusions

G. Organic anxiety syndrome
1. State of anxiety with normal consciousness
2. Absence of impaired intellectual ability, hallucinations, or delusions

III. Nursing process in organic mental disorders

A. Assessment
1. Evaluate for characteristic physiologic responses (see section I.C), such as:
    a. Possible hypoxic symptoms
    b. Possible metabolic disorder symptoms
    c. Possible toxic states or signs of infection
    d. Possible structural changes (e.g., atherosclerosis, neurofibrillary tangles symptoms)
    e. Possible vascular pathology symptoms
    f. Possible neurologic disease symptoms (motor deficits)

g. Self-care impairment related to confusional state (lack of eating, bowel and bladder incontinence)
h. Altered sleep pattern
i. Sensory impairment
2. Assess for behavioral responses, such as:
    a. Inattention to self-care and activities of daily living (ADLs)
    b. Apraxia (loss of ability to perform skills)
    c. Short attention span
    d. Exaggerated mannerisms
    e. Deterioration in social skills; withdrawal from social roles
    f. Confused behavior and agitation, especially in early morning (sunrise syndrome) and in evening (sundown syndrome)
    g. Confabulation: fabricated responses
    h. Perseveration: repeating a word or phrase over and over
3. Assess for characteristic cognitive responses, including:
    a. Disorientation to time, place, or person
    b. Deficits in memory and recall (especially short-term memory)
    c. Impaired intellectual functioning; difficulties in knowledge application, reasoning, problem solving
    d. Deficits in judgment (e.g., inappropriate social behavior, inability to decide courses of action)
    e. Difficulty sorting out sensory information; perceptual difficulties (agnosia)
4. Observe for such affective responses as:
    a. Emotional lability
    b. Inappropriate emotional responses
    c. Irritability, defensiveness
    d. Loss of interest, detachment (emotional dulling)
    e. Depression
    f. Suspicion

B. Analysis and nursing diagnoses
1. The nurse needs knowledge of the pathologic processes that result in impaired cognition and orientation.
2. Accurate analysis also requires knowledge of the normal aging process.
3. The nurse also needs to have empathy and persistence in intervening with impaired cognition and confusional states, especially in elderly patients.
4. Pertinent North American Nursing Diagnosis Association (NANDA) diagnoses can include:
    a. Altered Thought Processes
    b. Sensory-Perceptual Alteration
    c. Self-Care Deficit: Feeding, Toileting, Dressing, Grooming
    d. Impaired Communication: Verbal

   e.   Bowel Incontinence
   f.   Altered Urinary Elimination: Incontinence
   g.   Altered Role Performance
   h.   Altered Family Processes
C.   Planning and implementation
   1.   Provide emergency measures as necessary (e.g., for aspiration, asphyxia, injury from confused behavior or seizures); anticipate hazards and prevent injury.
   2.   Respond to underlying organic disease processes as indicated (e.g., hydration, antibiotics, vitamins, oxygenation).
   3.   Maintain fluid and electrolyte balance.
   4.   Maintain nutritional balance.
   5.   Promote structured elimination patterns; use disposable pants as needed to maintain dignity.
   6.   Promote rest by active daily schedule, avoiding hypnotics.
   7.   Minimize risk of cardiovascular problems (medication, diet, exercise, rest, stress management).
   8.   Monitor drugs and drug interactions; titrate medications carefully.
   9.   Facilitate the patient doing as much by self or with assistance as possible without frustration; be creative in ADL assistance or support.
   10.   Promote involvement or inclusion in ADLs; use positive reinforcement.
   11.   Decrease environmental stimuli and call the patient by name to focus attention; use short, clear messages.
   12.   Include the patient in family functions; support the patient and family in altered roles and inappropriate social behavior with community resources (e.g., support groups, day care, respite care).
   13.   Provide orienting information concerning time, place, person; use environmental supports such as clocks, calendars, and consistent routine, and sensory aids such as glasses or hearing aids, as needed.
   14.   Do not reinforce or agree with hallucinations and delusions as really occurring, but focus on feelings being indirectly expressed.
   15.   Do not approach the patient rapidly or use touch if irritable, agitated, or suspicious; use restraints minimally.
   16.   Support the patient's memory with reminders, structured environment, routines, orientation boards.
   17.   Support the patient in intellectual functions by avoiding stressful demands, supporting or limiting decision making, providing stimulation.
   18.   Assist in avoiding or limiting socially embarrassing situations; support the family in adjusting and accepting socially inappropriate incidents.

19. Reduce excessive stimuli, reduce pace, avoid procedures if the patient is agitated, make demands and communications simple.
20. Facilitate expression of feelings of loss or grief, frustration by the patient and family.
21. Maintain alertness to rapid shifts in emotion; do not approach the patient rapidly or use touch when the patient is agitated.
22. Use a nonjudgmental, empathic approach with the patient and family.

D. Evaluation
1. The patient exhibits improved cognition and sensory function.
2. The patient demonstrates improved ability to perform ADL.
3. The patient demonstrates improved communication ability.
4. The patient maintains adequate bowel and urinary elimination patterns.
5. The patient maintains adequate nutrition and fluid intake.
6. The patient exhibits improved socialization patterns.
7. The patient displays increased emotional stability.

Bibliography

Janosik, E. H., & Davies, E. L. (1987). *Psychiatric mental health nursing.* Boston: Jones & Bartlett.

Johnson, B. S. (1989). *Psychiatric-mental health nursing: Adaptation and growth* (2nd ed.). Philadelphia: J. B. Lippincott.

Stuart, G. W., & Sundeen, S. J. (1987). *Principles and practice of psychiatric nursing* (3rd ed.). St. Louis: C.V. Mosby.

Wilson, H. S., & Kneisl, C. R. (1988). *Psychiatric nursing* (3rd ed.). Menlo Park, CA: Addison-Wesley.

STUDY QUESTIONS

1. Which of the following statements regarding the clinical distinction between
psychotic and neurotic behavior is correct?
   a. A neurosis involves both disorientation and anxiety.
   b. A psychosis involves disorientation
   to time, place, and person.
   c. A neurosis is always accompanied by
   psychotic behavior.
   d. A functional disorder is an organic
   disorder.

2. A degenerative disorder of cognition primarily associated with age or metabolic
deterioration is known as
   a. dementia
   b. delirium
   c. psychosis
   d. neurosis

3. The most essential basic aspect of care
for persons with mental disorders is
   a. strict compliance with the medical
   regimen
   b. establishment of nurse–patient rapport
   c. constant vigil for suicide attempts
   d. administration of prescribed drug
   therapy

4. Basic psychologic assessment of level of
consciousness includes which of the following?
   a. cranial nerve 12 function
   b. cerebellar functioning
   c. anxiety and stress levels
   d. orientation to time, place, and
   person

5. In contrast to organic disorder, functional mental illness primarily results
from
   a. genetic endowment
   b. social milieu
   c. infection and inflammation
   d. degeneration of brain tissue

6. Which of the following medications is
used to combat secondary dementia related to an overdose of narcotics and in-
toxication?

   a. amphetamine sulfate (Benzedrine)
   b. naloxone hydrochloride (Narcan)
   c. dextroamphetamine (Dexedrine)
   d. caffeine sodium benzoate

7. Which of the following interventions is
most appropriate in a crisis situation, be
it of organic or functional origin?
   a. Encourage socialization.
   b. Support ego strengths.
   c. Meet all dependency needs.
   d. Initiate psychotherapy.

8. Which of the following organic conditions is well known for being exhibited
as delirium, especially in children?
   a. infection
   b. pernicious anemia
   c. hypothyroidism
   d. fever

9. Dementia is best defined as which of the
following?
   a. memory loss occurring as a natural
   consequence of aging
   b. poor judgment, especially in social
   relationships
   c. personal neglect in self-care
   d. loss of intellectual abilities sufficient
   to impair ability to perform ADLs

10. Which of the following characteristics
distinguishes delirium from dementia?
   a. progressive loss of consciousness
   b. abrupt disorientation with return to
   ADLs
   c. nonfluctuating levels of awareness
   d. memory loss and inappropriate social response

11. As an organic cognitive problem
emerges, a person's coping mechanism
will probably fit which of the following
characteristics?
   a. emergence of new coping methods
   b. display of anger or depression
   c. use of familiar patterns of responding to stress
   d. immediate regressive behaviors

12. Which of the following interventions is
of primary importance in working with
patients experiencing dementia?

    a. speaking to the patient with short words and simple sentences
    b. administering tranquilizers
    c. promoting increased exercise
    d. reinforcing the patient's thought patterns

ANSWER KEY

1. *Correct response: b*
   Psychosis involves disorientation to time, place, and person as well as other cognitive disorders.
   a. Neurosis is characterized by anxiety but not disorientation.
   c. Neuroses are not associated with psychoses.
   d. A functional disorder is nonorganic.
   Knowledge/Psychosocial/Assessment

2. *Correct response: a*
   Dementias are progressive, often associated with aging or an underlying metabolic or organic deterioration.
   b. Delirium is characterized by abrupt, spontaneous cognitive dysfunction with an underlying organic mental disorder.
   c and d. Psychosis and neurosis are psychologic diagnoses.
   Knowledge/Psychosocial/Assessment

3. *Correct response: b*
   Patient rapport, comfort, and trust are basic components of nursing care.
   a and d. These measures are aspects of a medical regimen.
   c. This may be appropriate for some patients but is not always essential for every patient with a mental disorder.
   Application/Safe care/Implementation

4. *Correct response: d*
   The initial and most basic assessment for altered level of consciousness is orientation.
   a, b, and c. These aspects are not associated with assessing level of consciousness.
   Application/Physiologic/Assessment

5. *Correct response: b*
   Functional mental illness is most commonly linked to social environment.
   a. Genetic endowment is associated with some disorders.
   c and d. Infection and inflammation and degeneration are commonly associated with organic mental disorders.
   Knowledge/Psychosocial/NA

6. *Correct response: b.*
   Narcan is a narcotic antagonist.
   a, c, and d. These drugs are indicated for other specific therapies.
   Application/Safe care/Implementation

7. *Correct response: d*
   Psychologic needs must be met first in order to attend to the crisis.
   a, b, and c. After meeting immediate psychologic needs, the nurse can consider these other aspects of care.
   Application/Safe care/Implementation

8. *Correct response: d*
   Both the very young and the elderly are vulnerable to hyperthermic conditions leading to delirium.
   a. Infection can occur in both adults and children.
   b and c. Pernicious anemia and hypothyroidism would be more common causes in adults.
   Comprehension/Physiologic/Analysis (Dx)

9. *Correct response: d*
   Self-care ability is an important measure of the progression of dementia.
   a. Loss of memory leading to dementia is not necessarily a natural consequence of age, but rather reflects underlying physical, metabolic, and pathologic processes.
   b and c. These effects typically accompany dementias but are not considered defining characteristics.
   Comprehension/Psychosocial/Analysis (Dx)

10. *Correct response: b*
    Abrupt disorientation with return to premorbid level of awareness and a self-care ability is a hallmark of delirium.
    a, c, and d. These characteristics are associated with dementias.
    Knowledge/Psychosocial/Assessment

11. *Correct response: c*
    Most persons will fall back on their personal, familiar response patterns to stress.

a. New and unfamiliar methods become impossible for persons with progressive dementia.
b. Anger and depression are possible but are not usual ways of coping.
d. Regressive behaviors are more commonly associated with late stages of dementia.

Analysis/Psychosocial/Assessment

12. *Correct response: a*

Short sentences and simple words minimize patient confusion and enhance communication.

b. Tranquilizers generally are not appropriate except to treat other concurrent conditions.
c. Exercise may be important for some patients, but it is not a primary consideration in dealing with dementia.
d. Reality orientation, rather than feeding into the patient's altered thought patterns, is an important goal.

Application/Safe care/Implementation

Treatment Modalities: Crisis Intervention

I. Overview

A. Definitions

1. A crisis is a threatening situation in which usual problem-solving or decision-making methods are not adequate to cope adaptively.
2. Crisis situations are life transitions or stressful events that are time-limited (up to 6 weeks).

B. Types of crises

1. Developmental-maturational crises include:
    a. Birth of a child
    b. Beginning school
    c. Puberty
    d. Old age

    2. Developmental-transitional crises include:
        a. Birth of siblings
        b. Marriage
        c. Death of significant other
    3. Situational-victim crises include:
        a. Loss of job, divorce
        b. Rape
        c. Murder
        d. Incest
    4. Situational-disaster crises (also called adventitious crises) include:
        a. Tornadoes
        b. Earthquakes
        c. Fires
        d. Airplane crashes

C. Sequence of crisis development
    1. The precrisis period is marked by:
        a. Emotional equilibrium
        b. Effective coping mechanisms
    2. Features of the crisis period include:
        a. Upset in steady state
        b. Rise in tension
        c. Usual coping skills not successful
    3. The postcrisis period involves:
        a. Return to (or increase or decrease in) usual level of functioning
        b. Resolution of crisis

D. Loss and the grieving process
    1. Crisis intervention theory emerged from research on the grieving process.
    2. Death is a universal experience anticipated with anxiety.
    3. Grieving is an experience related to loss of a loved one or a valued object, ideal, position, or status.
    4. Phases of grieving include:
        a. First phase: shock and disbelief
        b. Second phase: developing awareness of loss and emotional pain
        c. Third phase: resolution, reorganization (takes up to 2 years)
    5. Indicators of pathologic mourning include:
        a. Inability to experience or express painful feelings about loss
        b. Failure to acknowledge and accept loss
        c. Anniversary reactions: becoming depressed on anniversary dates of loss
        d. Prolonged and serious alterations in social adjustment
        e. Development of agitated depression or suicidality

E. **Balancing factors affecting equilibrium**
   1. Perception of the event involves:
       a. How crisis event is appraised
       b. Coping behaviors
   2. Situational supports include:
       a. Persons on whom the person in crisis can depend
       b. Other resources (e.g., money, housing, social services)
   3. Coping skills depend on:
       a. Use of defense mechanisms (see Chapter 3 for a review of defense mechanisms)
       b. Handling of previous crises
       c. Problem-solving ability
       d. Current number of stressors in life

F. **Characteristics of crisis situations and crisis intervention**
   1. Crisis situations may produce such physiologic and psychologic effects as:
       a. Physiologic symptoms of anxiety: diarrhea, dizziness, shortness of breath, palpitations
       b. Sleep disturbances
       c. Restlessness, lack of concentration
       d. Irritability, outbursts of anger
       e. Agitation, crying
       f. Inability to make decisions
       g. Paranoid thoughts, feelings of isolation
       h. Suicidal or homicidal ideation
   2. Because a patient in crisis feels overwhelmed and unable to cope, effective crisis intervention must build on the patient's existing strengths and resources.

II. **Disorders related to unresolved crises**

A. **Adjustment disorder**
   1. Description: maladaptive reaction to an identifiable psychosocial stressor occurring within 3 months of the stressor's onset and persisting for no more than 6 months
   2. Reaction to the stressor is excessive and involves impaired social or occupational functioning.
   3. Types of adjustment disorders include:
       a. Adjustment disorder with depressed mood
       b. Adjustment disorder with anxious mood
       c. Adjustment disorder with mixed emotional features
       d. Adjustment disorder with disturbances of conduct
       e. Adjustment disorder with work or academic inhibition
       f. Adjustment disorder with withdrawal

B. **Post-traumatic stress syndrome (also see Chapter 3)**
   1. This disorder develops after a psychologically traumatic event (e.g., war, famine, natural disaster, physical attack, rape).

2. Characteristic symptoms include:
   a. Reexperiencing of traumatic event
   b. Recurrent, distressing dreams of event
   c. Variety of autonomic, depressed, or anxious symptoms
   d. Difficulty participating in external world

III. Nursing process in crisis intervention

A. Assessment

1. Identify the precipitating event and explore:
   a. Circumstances that brought on the crisis
   b. The event's chronologic sequence
   c. Factors that affect the patient's ability to solve the crisis
2. Explore the patient's perception of the crisis event, including:
   a. Themes and memories that reveal the meaning of the crisis to the patient
   b. Underlying needs that are threatened by the crisis
   c. Degree of disruption caused by the crisis
3. Assess support systems, including:
   a. Living situation (i.e., living alone or with family or friends)
   b. Persons available to help the patient
   c. Other support systems or resources (e.g., financial, religious, social)
4. Assess coping skills, covering:
   a. How the patient has handled similar crises in the past
   b. Personal strengths and weaknesses
   c. Adaptive defense mechanisms
   d. Coping skill deficits

B. Analysis and nursing diagnoses

1. The nurse should be aware of potential crises in various nursing practice areas, including:
   a. Maternal–child: birth of premature infant, stillborn infant, birth anomalies
   b. Pediatrics: onset of a serious illness, chronic or debilitating illnesses, severe accidents, a dying child
   c. Medical–surgical: learning about a serious diagnosis, debilitating illness, loss of body part or function, death and dying
   d. Gerontology: cumulative losses, debilitating illness, dependency, nursing home placement
   e. Emergency: physical trauma, acute illness, rape, death
   f. Psychiatry: being hospitalized with a psychiatric disorder, life stressors for the chronically mentally ill, suicidality
2. Pertinent North American Nursing Diagnosis Association (NANDA) diagnoses can include:
   a. Ineffective Individual Coping
      (1) Related to traumatic personal event

           (2)   Related to loss of significant other (or other losses)

           (3)   Related to inability to cope with stress

    b.   Altered Family Process

           (1)   Related to inability to deal with family transitions

           (2)   Related to geographic relocation

           (3)   Related to grief

C. Planning and implementation

1. Use effective problem-solving processes with the patient, including:

    a.   Assisting him or her to gain understanding of the crisis; breaking crisis down into component problems

    b.   Helping correct misperceptions about the crisis

    c.   Promoting expression of feelings

    d.   Supporting adaptive defense mechanisms through reinforcement

    e.   Exploring options for resolution of crisis; giving suggestions as needed

2. Intervene in any plans for suicide or homicide by:

    a.   Taking warning signs seriously

    b.   Determining the concreteness of the plan (a concrete plan increases the likelihood of an attempt)

    c.   Removing dangerous and potentially lethal materials or objects where possible

    d.   Placing the patient in a safe, protective environment and monitoring closely and consistently or mobilizing support

    e.   Communicating your presence and desire to protect the patient from harming himself or herself or others

    f.   Encouraging the patient to talk about stressors; feelings of pain, anger, and anguish; and suicide or homicide plans

    g.   Listening empathically

    h.   Reinforcing the patient's desire to resolve problems, to live

    i.   Referring the patient for follow-up treatment

3. Raise the patient's self esteem by:

    a.   Acknowledging his or her strengths

    b.   Empathizing with the patient and his or her situation

    c.   Mobilizing the patient to constructive actions

    d.   Offering yourself in an active way; staying with the patient, expressing caring and concern

4. Mobilize the patient's support systems by:

    a.   Helping him or her contact family or friends who will be supportive

    b.   Referring him or her to appropriate social or community services

5. Provide anticipatory guidance and follow-up, including:

    a.   Reviewing various consequences for each possible solution

b. Providing the opportunity to rehearse what might be done now and in future crises
c. Providing support for a patient anticipating a potentially stressful situation (e.g., surgery, childbirth)
d. Providing support for a patient who has experienced a stressful event (e.g., rape, child abuse, natural disaster)

D. **Evaluation**
1. The patient demonstrates absence of presenting crisis behavior: physiologic, behavioral, cognitive, affective.
2. The patient exhibits return to precrisis state or improved situation or behavior.

Bibliography

Janosik, E. H., & Davies, E. L. (1987). *Psychiatric mental health nursing.* Boston: Jones & Bartlett.

Johnson, B. S. (1989). *Psychiatric-mental health nursing: Adaptation and growth* (2nd ed.). Philadelphia: J. B. Lippincott.

Stuart, G. W., & Sundeen, S. J. (1987). *Principles and practice of psychiatric nursing* (3rd ed.). St. Louis: C. V. Mosby.

Wilson, H. S., & Kneisl, C. R. (1988). *Psychiatric nursing* (3rd ed.). Menlo Park, CA: Addison-Wesley.

STUDY QUESTIONS

1. After a happy childhood, Sally, aged 13, is having a difficult adolescence. She grew 5 inches in the last year and developed rather large breasts. One day after some boys in her class teased and intimidated her, Sally went to the school nurse in tears. Sally is so affected by the teasing and intimidation that she starts to withdraw and perform less effectively in her school work. Based on this information, the school nurse would conclude that Sally is experiencing what type of crisis?
   a. developmental-maturational
   b. developmental-transitional
   c. situational-victim
   d. combination of situational and developmental

2. What is the first step the school nurse should take?
   a. Call Sally's mother.
   b. Have Sally tell in detail what happened.
   c. Ask Sally who her best friends are.
   d. Take Sally's temperature and pulse.

3. As Sally talks about the events that precipitated her crisis, the nurse learns that she is a lonely girl with few friends. Which of the following actions would be most appropriate for the nurse to take at this time?
   a. Suggest that Sally transfer to another nearby school.
   b. Suggest that Sally ask the boys in her class to stop teasing her.
   c. Suggest that Sally volunteer to help others.
   d. Suggest that Sally visit the nurse on a regular basis.

4. Which of the following questions would best help the nurse to clarify Sally's perception of the crisis event?
   a. "Do you know the boys who teased you?"
   b. "Have you noticed that other girls get teased also?"
   c. "Can you tell me what happened first?"

   d. "Do you think the boys meant to hurt your feelings?"

5. As Sally comes to trust the nurse, which of the following nursing actions most likely would enhance Sally's ability to deal with her situation?
   a. Explore ways to deal with teasing of classmates.
   b. Talk to the school principal about the teasing.
   c. Discuss aspects of adolescent development.
   d. Express empathy for the trauma Sally has experienced.

6. Dawn, aged 17, was raped by a young man in her neighborhood. She is in the Emergency Room for treatment and requires laboratory tests. After the procedures are completed, a psychiatric clinical nurse specialist takes Dawn into the conference room for rape counseling. Implementing a system of routine counseling for a rape victim represents
   a. assessment
   b. anticipatory crisis intervention
   c. empathic concern
   d. unwarranted intrusion

7. During the assessment process, which of the following actions would be appropriate?
   a. Have Dawn recount the events of the rape.
   b. Encourage Dawn to talk about her early childhood.
   c. Allow Dawn to call her boyfriend.
   d. Ask Dawn to describe the rapist.

8. Dawn expresses her belief that the rape was her fault because she walked down the alley on her way to school. Which of the following actions should the nurse take to address Dawn's perception?
   a. Ask Dawn what other behaviors may have contributed to the rape.
   b. Suggest that Dawn walk to school with a group of classmates.
   c. Agree that taking the alley to school is risky behavior.

    d. Emphasize that the rapist, not Dawn, is responsible for the rape.

9. Dawn wants to go home from the Emergency Room by herself. What would be the best way for the nurse to respond to Dawn's wish?

    a. Ask Dawn how she will get home.

    b. Call a family member for Dawn before she leaves.

    c. Drive Dawn home herself.

    d. Let Dawn do as she wishes.

10. Mr. Thomas, aged 33, has a chronic mental illness. He lives in a halfway house where meals and medications are provided. Each day he takes the bus 5 miles to his job as an assistant janitor for a large apartment building. One day, Mr. Thomas loses his wallet on the bus. He becomes extremely upset, gets off the bus, and starts to walk back to the halfway house. It starts to snow heavily, and he becomes confused about directions and gets lost. He finally wanders into a store and asks the owner to call the police. Based on this information, the nurse could make which of the following analyses about Tom?

    a. He has a deficit in coping skills that predisposes him to crises.

    b. He should not be allowed to travel on his own via public transportation.

    c. He is not in crisis because he is chronically mentally ill.

    d. He is a victim of circumstances.

11. In the above scenario, which of Tom's actions indicates a coping strength?

    a. deciding to walk home

    b. not telling anyone about the lost wallet

    c. becoming extremely upset about the lost wallet

    d. calling the police

ANSWER KEY

1. **Correct response: d**
   Adolescence presents a time of crisis for Sally; having the boys in her class teasing her adds a situational-victim type of crisis.
   a and c. Although these are also correct, they are incomplete answers.
   b. Transitional crises refer to major transitions such as marriage and the birth of a child.
   Comprehension/Psychosocial/Assessment

2. **Correct response: b**
   The first step in crisis intervention is to obtain the patient's perception of the crisis event.
   a and c. These refer to situational supports, which are mobilized later in the intervention process.
   d. There are no physiologic indicators pointing to the need for this action.
   Application/Psychosocial/Assessment

3. **Correct response: d**
   By becoming directly available to Sally, the nurse raises Sally's self-esteem. The nurse becomes involved in an active way, which is appropriate in crisis intervention.
   a, b, and c. These responses avoid direct involvement with the patient in crisis.
   Analysis/Psychosocial/Implementation

4. **Correct response: c**
   Placing the events in chronologic sequence is helpful in clarifying what happened.
   a, b, and d. These are less useful questions and also are closed-ended. It would be better to help Sally get started with open-ended questions.
   Application/Psychosocial/Assessment

5. **Correct response: a**
   Once trust has developed, the nurse can help Sally think of alternative coping skills to deal with the problems she encounters.
   b. Through this action, the nurse would be attempting to solve the problem for Sally rather than helping Sally learn new coping skills.
   c. This action addresses understanding rather than problem solving.
   d. Although empathy is very important, it is used for building trust and rapport and does not address problem solving.
   Analysis/Psychosocial/Implementation

6. **Correct response: b**
   Anticipatory guidance is part of the crisis intervention model. Certain stressful events, such as rape, make a person more vulnerable to crisis. Counseling at the time of the stressful event can strengthen the patient's coping skills and prevent a full-blown crisis from occurring.
   a, c, and d. These responses do not describe the intervention.
   Comprehension/Health promotion/Implementation

7. **Correct response: a**
   Crisis intervention begins with having the patient talk about the precipitating event in detail. In this way, the nurse can assess how Dawn perceives the event.
   b. Early childhood exploration is not a usual component of crisis intervention.
   c and d. These aspects might be addressed later on in the counseling session.
   Application/Psychosocial/Assessment

8. **Correct response: d**
   Through exploring the precipitating events, the nurse observes for and corrects apparent misperceptions about the event. In this case, Dawn sees the rape as her fault. The nurse gives Dawn a more realistic perception.
   a, b, and c. These actions lay the re-

sponsibility for the rape on Dawn.
Application/Psychosocial/Implementation

9. *Correct response: b*
Crisis intervention should mobilize the patient's support system. By offering to call the family, the nurse remains involved in an active way.

    a and d. The patient needs the support of family or friends after experiencing such a traumatic event.

    c. This service would be better provided by a family member, a volunteer, or even the police.
Application/Safe care/Implementation

10. *Correct response: a*
Chronically mentally ill patients like Tom are vulnerable to crises because their coping skills are less adaptive.

When he lost his wallet, he panicked and got off the bus.

    b. Tom has been able to handle the bus trip on a regular basis, and continued independence should be encouraged.

    c. Just the opposite is true; chronically mentally ill patients are very vulnerable to crises.

    d. Tom could have handled things differently.
Analysis/Psychosocial/Analysis (Dx)

11. *Correct response: d*
By calling the police, Tom demonstrated sufficient understanding of his situation to know that he needed help. He contacted an appropriate social institution to mobilize support on his behalf.

    a, b, and c. These are all indicators of poor problem-solving skills.
Application/Psychosocial/Assessment

Treatment Modalities:

Group Therapy

I. Overview
A. Definitions
1. Group: a social system with interdependent members interacting reciprocally
   a. Average size is six to 12 members (small groups).
   b. Members usually have something in common.
2. Group dynamics: the interactions and relationships existing within the group

B. Stages of group development
1. Most groups proceed through fairly well-anticipated phases:
   a. Orientation phase (beginning stage)
   b. Working phase (middle stage)
   c. Termination phase (ending stage)
2. Expected patient behaviors in the *orientation phase* include:
   a. High anxiety

        b.   Hesitancy, uncertainty

        c.   Unclear contract expectations

        d.   Superficial sharing; focus on self

        e.   Testing of therapist and other group members

  3.   Expected patient behaviors in the *working phase* include:

        a.   Increased self-disclosure

        b.   Developing sense of group feeling, evolving concern for other members

        c.   Working on problems or concerns

        d.   Possible in-depth exploration of a topic or problem

  4.   Expected patient behaviors during the *termination phase* include:

        a.   Expression of varying feelings about termination (e.g., anger, sadness, joy, rejection)

        b.   Possible increased testing of therapist

        c.   Possible sense of loneliness or fear

C. **Group dynamics**

  1.   Group content refers to verbal communication among members.

  2.   Group process refers to what occurs within the group, including:

        a.   Nonverbal communication among members

        b.   Relationships or interchanges among members

        c.   Body language, gestures

        d.   Seating arrangements

        e.   Speaking patterns or tones

        f.   Group themes: may be expressed overtly or covertly

  3.   Group cohesiveness refers to the sense of belonging, of unity, of ''groupness''; it involves:

        a.   Loyalty and allegiance to the group

        b.   High degree of participation and sharing among members

        c.   Nonjudgmental attitudes among members

        d.   Maintenance of group norms

        e.   High member attendance and low dropout rate

        f.   High tolerance for conflict or disagreement

        g.   Effective problem-solving mechanisms

        h.   Sense of group togetherness

  4.   Group norms refer to implicit or explicit rules defining members' behavior; types include:

        a.   Productive norms, which enhance cohesiveness (e.g., all members' opinions respected, only one person speaks at a time)

        b.   Nonproductive norms, which inhibit cohesiveness (e.g., no disagreements allowed, absenteeism or tardiness accepted)

  5.   Group roles refer to the parts various members play within the group, including:

        a.   Initiator: suggests innovative ideas, starts the interactions

        b.   Coordinator: organizes and integrates

      c.   Evaluator: appraises group performance
      d.   Information-seeker: elicits facts
      e.   Gatekeeper: screens input and maintains open communication
      f.   Encourager: praises and accepts
      g.   Harmonizer: maintains peace through compromise, alternatives
      h.   Commentator: processes the group interaction
      i.   Blocker: inhibits the group's advancement
      j.   Recognition-seeker: self-aggrandizes
      k.   Monopolizer: controls by endless talking
      l.   Self-confessor: discloses personal information inappropriately

6. Leadership refers to both the therapist's and members' responsibilities for guiding the group; types of small group leadership include (Table 13–1):
      a.   Authoritarian
      b.   Democratic
      c.   Laissez-faire

7. Generally, a group functions best when leadership is shared among members, particularly during the middle stage (working phase).

8. Power refers to the ability to influence others. A successful group power structure helps all members meet their needs. Some groups may experience ongoing realignment or struggles for power.

D. Advantages and disadvantages of group therapy
1. Advantages include:
      a.   Helps group members learn that their problems are not unique
      b.   Promotes interpersonal relationships through actual participation
      c.   Facilitates group members' participation in problem solving of personal and others' problems
      d.   Provides multiple sources of feedback and reality testing
2. Disadvantages include:
      a.   Reduces individual attention from the leader
      b.   Necessitates reduced intensity of focus on or support for an individual's problems or pain
      c.   May create a lack of confidence in confidentiality

E. Characteristics of groups (especially therapy groups)
1. In cohesive groups:
      a.   Group norms are maintained (e.g., attendance is high and members arrive on time).
      b.   Trust has been established.

TABLE 13–1.
Common Leadership Styles

STYLE	CHARACTERISTICS

Authoritarian	The leader
	    Exerts total control
	    Makes the decisions, establishes policies, and decides goals and purposes.
	    Discourages communication and sharing among members; all communication is directed to the leader
	    Is task-oriented
	Group members
	    May be frustrated and angry
	    Act-out by scapegoating or exhibiting passive-aggressive behavior
	The group atmosphere generally is tense.
	This style may be effective for large groups and when quick decisions are needed.

Democratic	The leader
	    Encourages member involvement and collaboration
	    Promotes group cohesiveness and the development of productive norms
	    Facilitates individual input and growth
	    Promotes open communication
	Group members generally like the group.
	The atmosphere tends to be more comfortable.

Laissez-faire	The leader
	    Functions as a consultant/resource person
	    Provides minimal direction
	    Promotes minimal interpersonal interactions among members
	Group members
	    May feel lost without directions
	    May be disorganized
	    May be apathetic
	    Tend to be self-focused
	Productivity is reduced.
	The atmosphere is haphazard.
	This style may be effective for groups of highly self-directed persons.

    c.   Participation is high and on a deep-feeling level.
    d.   Commitment or loyalty to the group increases over time; members stay in group.
    e.   Mutual support is offered.
    f.   Member-to-member influence is present.
    g.   Productivity ("work") is evident.
    h.   Group concerns ("we") become more pronounced than individual concerns.

       i.   Leadership usually is democratic and shared to some extent among members.

    2. In noncohesive groups:

       a.   Group norms are lacking or violated (e.g., absenteeism, tardiness).

       b.   There is lack of trust, uncertainty or suspicion among members.

       c.   Participation is minimal and sporadic.

       d.   There is poor loyalty to the group, individual competition among members, and a high dropout rate.

       e.   There is a lack of interpersonal concern among members.

       f.   There is member-to-member criticism, competition.

       g.   Productivity and work achievement are lacking.

       h.   There are pronounced individual concerns ("I") as compared to those of the group.

       i.   There is usually an autocratic or very laissez-faire leadership style; therapist-dominated.

II. Types of groups

A. Therapy or support groups

    1. *Group psychotherapy* may focus on:

       a.   Personality reconstruction

       b.   Insight, self-awareness

       c.   Remotivation

       d.   Problem solving

       e.   Reeducation

       f.   Support

    2. *Therapeutic (primary prevention, crisis intervention) groups* may provide:

       a.   Prevention

       b.   Education

       c.   Support

    3. *Self-help groups* (led by group members) may be aimed at providing:

       a.   Behavioral improvement

       b.   Stress reduction

       c.   Self-esteem, social integration maintenance

B. Other types of groups

    1. *Task-oriented groups* (e.g., committees) focus on:

       a.   Performance of specific job or assignment

       b.   Achievement of mission or goals for a larger group

    2. *Teaching–learning groups* focus on:

       a.   Skill acquisition

       b.   Information sharing

    3. *Social groups* convene for:

       a.   Recreation, relaxation

   b. Fun, pleasure

   c. Companionship

   d. Satisfaction, acquisition of social skills

III. Nursing process in group therapy

 A. **Assessment**

  1. Evaluate individual patients' behavior in the group context.

  2. Assess verbal content in the group setting.

  3. Assess group processes, noting:

   a. Where members sit

   b. Who talks with whom and about what

   c. Tones of voice used by members

   d. Response to group norms

   e. Congruence of verbal content and process

   f. Roles

   g. Evolution of group cohesiveness

 B. **Analysis and nursing diagnoses**

  1. Recognize the effects of behavior of the group and yourself on group members.

  2. Apply knowledge of group dynamics.

  3. Relevant North American Nursing Diagnosis Association (NANDA) diagnoses may include:

   a. Ineffective Individual Coping

   b. Impaired Social Interaction

   c. Anxiety

   d. Impaired Adjustment

   e. Dysfunctional Grieving

 C. **Planning and implementation**

  1. During the *orientation phase:*

   a. Be directive and active.

   b. Establish contract for meetings and relationships.

   c. Promote production norms and group cohesiveness.

   d. Encourage open communication and exploration of feelings and ideas.

   e. Listen, observe, and give therapeutic feedback.

   f. Comment on behavior that enhances or hinders constructive group process.

   g. Assist individual members and the group to evaluate behaviors.

  2. During the *working phase:*

   a. Assume the roles of consultant and facilitator.

   b. Recognize conflicts; label them and explore meanings.

   c. Assist the group to deal constructively with conflicts and problems.

   d. Assist the group to examine the impact of subgroups, scapegoating, absenteeism, and passive-aggressive behavior, as applicable.

3. During the *termination phase:*
    a. Assume a more direct, supportive role.
    b. Assist members to verbalize and explore feelings and thoughts about termination.
    c. Encourage evaluation of group and individual members' progress.
    d. Provide adequate time for members to deal with termination.
    e. Refer those whose needs were unmet by the group for further evaluation and care, as appropriate.

D. **Evaluation**
    1. Group
        a. The group exhibits good cohesiveness; members demonstrate shared allegiance and responsibility to the group.
        b. Norms are productive and enhance members' emotional development.
        c. Group maintenance and group task roles are predominant.
        d. Communication occurs among members and not just between the leader and members.
        e. Leadership is shared among members.
        f. Members work together as a team to reach goals and to resolve problems and conflicts.
        g. Termination occurs with a sense of accomplishment.
    2. Individual
        a. The patient demonstrates improved communication ability.
        b. The patient exhibits improved problem-solving skills.
        c. The patient reports improved coping with life issues.

Bibliography

Janosik, E. H., & Davies, E. L. (1987). *Psychiatric mental health nursing.* Boston: Jones & Bartlett.

Johnson, B. S. (1989). *Psychiatric-mental health nursing: Adaptation and growth* (2nd ed.). Philadelphia: J. B. Lippincott.

Stuart, G. W., & Sundeen, S. J. (1987). *Principles and practice of psychiatric nursing* (3rd ed.). St. Louis: C. V. Mosby.

Wilson, H. S., & Kneisl, C. R. (1988). *Psychiatric nursing* (3rd ed.). Menlo Park, CA: Addison-Wesley.

STUDY QUESTIONS

1. During a community meeting on an in-patient psychiatric unit, the nurse is having difficulty getting the members to take their seats and settle down. The nurse asks Mr. Guha, the community president (a patient elected by his peers), to start the meeting. Not 5 minutes into the meeting, a patient from one side of the room shouts to another patient on the other side of the room, "Can I have a cigarette?" The nurse should best deal with this situation by
   a. telling Mr. Guha to proceed
   b. asking the group to examine what has just happened
   c. apologizing to Mr. Guha
   d. ignoring the interaction

2. The appropriate intervention in the above situation is based on the nurse's plan to improve
   a. the group environment
   b. member retention
   c. interpersonal relationships among members
   d. members' decision-making abilities

3. Based on a nursing needs assessment revealing that parents in a clinic have misconceptions about child development that affect their ability to discipline, the nurse decides to form a teaching–learning group. The nurse chose a teaching–learning group over a support group because the focus should be on
   a. information, not feelings
   b. socialization, not insight
   c. insight, not information
   d. feelings, not socialization

4. A group of 15 neighbors meet monthly to promote a safer neighborhood. Membership consists of both male and female adults, and the meeting place rotates among members' homes. The group had agreed to meet the first Monday of each month at 7:00 PM. The nurse was asked to attend tonight's meeting as a consultant. By 7:00 PM, only three members had arrived; at 7:30 PM, one more person arrived. Mary, the group leader, says, "We've wasted 30 minutes; we should get started." James, another member, says, "It's important that everybody be here with facts that all of us need to hear." Mary continues, "What are we supposed to do? We can't make people come to this meeting. I could be at home doing my work. I don't have any more time to waste. Either we get started or I'm going to leave." James looks confused and hurt. Based on this information, the nurse would form which of the following impressions about the group?
   a. There are no norms.
   b. The norms are nonproductive.
   c. There are norms but they are not clearly stated.
   d. The norms are productive.

5. This group is characteristic of a
   a. task-directed group
   b. socialization group
   c. insight-oriented group
   d. teaching–learning group

6. This group is not cohesive because it
   a. doesn't have a designated leader
   b. has no group content
   c. has no group loyalty
   d. has no gatekeeper

7. In addition to the gatekeeper role, what other role is apparent in this group?
   a. blocker
   b. commentator
   c. evaluator
   d. harmonizer

8. After Mary's last statement, the nurse says, "From what I'm hearing, everybody that should be here isn't, and these absences, plus the waiting, are causing a lot of frustration." What is the purpose of this statement?
   a. to focus on group content
   b. to process the group
   c. to clarify group norms
   d. to provide an example of self-disclosure

9. John leads a group of adolescent boys in a biweekly meeting. He provides strong direction and discourages communication among group members. This leadership style is characterized as
   a. democratic leadership
   b. laissez-faire leadership
   c. authoritarian leadership
   d. distributed leadership

10. In John's group, members would most likely:
    a. be confused
    b. form a cohesive bond
    c. scapegoat another member
    d. demonstrate poor productivity

11. To determine this group's effectiveness, the nurse would do all of the following *except*
    a. Measure group members' participation in problem solving.
    b. Obtain only the leader's opinion.
    c. Observe group members' flow of communication.
    d. Look at the group's strategies for resolving conflict.

12. Which of the following reasons for a treatment team on an inpatient psychiatric unit to establish ward meetings would be appropriate?
    a. to provide an arena for the clients' complaints
    b. to promote involvement in ward management
    c. to address staff members' concerns
    d. to focus on survival on the outside

13. The purpose of screening candidates for group therapy is to determine
    a. friendliness
    b. sociability
    c. motivation
    d. intelligence

ANSWER KEY

1. *Correct response: b*
    Assisting the group to look at its behavior focuses members on the exploration, the analysis and the resolution of disruptive interpersonal relationships.
    a, c, and d. These actions would hinder group development.
    Application/Psychosocial/Implementation

2. *Correct response: c*
    The problem exemplified in this situation is a disruptive interpersonal relationship. Therefore, the plan has to address this problem.
    a, b, and d. None of these goals are relevant to the problem.
    Analysis/Psychosocial/Planning

3. *Correct response: a*
    These parents need didactic information to correct their misperceptions about child development.
    b, c, and d. There is no indication from this example that a support group or an insight-oriented group would be needed.
    Comprehension/Health promotion/Planning

4. *Correct response: b*
    This group is operating under nonproductive norms, which promote absenteeism.
    a, c, and d. This group has both explicit and implicit norms. There are explicit rules about meeting place and time, but implicit rules about absenteeism.
    Analysis/Psychosocial/Assessment

5. *Correct response: a*
    This group's purpose is promotion of a safer neighborhood.
    b, c, and d. The purpose isn't promotion of effective social skills, development of personal insight, or dis-

semination of factual information, respectively.
    Comprehension/Psychosocial/Assessment

6. *Correct response: c*
    Group loyalty, a measure of group cohesiveness, is not evident in this group, in which absenteeism is high and group participation is minimal.
    a, b, and d. These factors are not used to measure group cohesiveness.
    Analysis/Psychosocial/Assessment

7. *Correct response: a*
    Mary has assumed the role of blocker.
    b. No one has commented on the group process (commentator).
    c. No member has evaluated the group's performance (evaluator).
    d. No one has attempted to maintain peace (harmonizer).
    Analysis/Psychosocial/Assessment

8. *Correct response: b*
    This statement describes the group behavior on both a verbal and a nonverbal level and offers the group an opportunity to examine its behavior.
    a. The nurse's statement doesn't deal with group content—verbal communication.
    c. The nurse's statement doesn't address group norms—rules clarification.
    d. The nurse's statement doesn't involve self-disclosure—the revealing of personal information.
    Comprehension/Health promotion/ Implementation

9. *Correct response: c*
    An authoritarian leadership style involves exerting complete and total control over group members.
    a, b, and d. None of these leadership styles involves the type of control described in the scenario.
    Comprehension/Psychosocial/Assessment

10. *Correct response: c*

    In this scenario, group members likely would become frustrated and angry. Scapegoating provides one way of acting-out this frustration and anger.

    a, b, and d. These would not be expected responses in the scenario described.

    Comprehension/Psychosocial/Evaluation

11. *Correct response: b*

    Talking only to the authorized leader would give the nurse a skewed picture of the group.

    a, c, and d. All of these actions would help provide a more comprehensive and accurate picture of the group's effectiveness.

    Application/Psychosocial/Evaluation

12. *Correct response: b*

    Community meetings are designed to increase patients' involvement in the everyday management of their living environment.

    a, c, and d. Although these aims can be components of the community meetings, none is the primary purpose of holding the meetings.

    Knowledge/Psychosocial/Implementation

13. *Correct response: c*

    The candidate's motivation for group therapy is of utmost importance to the success he will experience in the group.

    a, b, and d. None of these are typical screening criteria.

    Knowledge/Psychosocial/Assessment

Treatment Modalities:
Family Therapy

I. Overview

A. Definitions

1. Family: a group of people living in one household who have emotional attachment, regular interaction, and shared concerns and responsibilities

2. Types of families:
   a. Traditional, nuclear family: married couple and their child or children by birth or adoption
   b. Single-parent family: lone parent and child or children by birth or adoption
   c. Blended family: married or nonmarried couple, one or both of whom were married previously, and his, her, or their child or children
   d. Alternative family: persons with or without blood or marital ties who live together to achieve common goals

3.   System: a set of elements that have reciprocal interactions or relationships among themselves; types and associated concepts include:
   a.   Suprasystem: a bigger system in which the family system functions (e.g., church, school, neighborhood, cultural group)
   b.   Subsystem: smaller subsets of the family system (e.g., siblings, parents, parent–child, intergenerational)
   c.   Boundaries: parameters defining who is inside and outside the system and the rules governing the system; may be open, closed, or diffused or unclear
   d.   Homeostasis: maintenance of system continuity, constancy, equilibrium
   e.   Synergy: cooperative action among members of a system such that the whole is greater than the sum of the parts (e.g., greater results are possible through family unity than through just individual members' efforts)

B.   Family systems
   1.   In a family, all members operate to maintain characteristic behavior, roles, and symptoms.
   2.   Relationships are characterized by a continuous cycle of interaction (circular cause-and-effect, not linear cause-and-effect).
   3.   Change in any part of the family system creates change in all other parts and in the whole system.
   4.   A person's family system is likely the most emotionally intense of all the systems in which he is involved.
   5.   Coalitions (e.g., dyad between two people) formed among members of the system may become problematic. For example, an intergenerational dyad may hinder intragenerational communication.
   6.   Triangles also may become problematic; examples include:
      a.   Three people
      b.   Two people and an issue
      c.   Two people and a group
   7.   Inappropriate distribution of power within the family also can create problems.

C.   Developmental issues of families
   1.   Phases of family development—particularly pertinent to traditional nuclear and blended families—include:
      a.   Coupling or marriage
      b.   Childbearing
      c.   Preschool-age children
      d.   School-age children
      e.   Teenage children

        f.   Launching children

        g.   Middle age

        h.   Aging family members

   2.   Developmental tasks of family systems include:

        a.   Physical maintenance: food, shelter, clothing

        b.   Physical and emotional resource allocation: expenses, goods, space, emotional support

        c.   Division of labor: financial, household management, child rearing

        d.   Socialization of members: physical, emotional, social, spiritual guidelines or rules

        e.   Entry and release of members: birth, adoption, moving out, visitation, living-in

        f.   Order: conformity to family or societal rules, standards, and norms

        g.   Interaction with larger systems: interface with church, school, neighborhood, society

        h.   Motivation and morale: guiding philosophy, family loyalty, reinforcement and rewards, traditions

D.   Communication in families

   1.   In family systems, important communication occurs on both verbal and nonverbal levels.

   2.   Verbal communication (e.g., who talks to whom, what is said, how something is said) helps define relationships within the system.

   3.   Nonverbal communication (e.g., body language, gestures, tone of voice, seating arrangements, timing of verbal feedback) helps define relationships within the system.

   4.   In good family communication, family members on a verbal and nonverbal level openly encourage clear, direct discussion of issues and feelings.

   5.   In maladaptive family communication, family members on a verbal and nonverbal level discourage open discussion of issues and feelings; both the message and the target of the message are unclear and confusing.

   6.   Pathologic communication patterns include:

        a.   Incongruence: relaying two conflicting messages at the same time (e.g., verbal and nonverbal messages do not match)

        b.   Double-bind: an incongruent message wherein the recipient is a victim and cannot "win" (e.g., "Do what I tell you—Be more independent.")

E.   Basic concepts: the individual in families

   1.   Individuation (the process of differentiating oneself, developing autonomy) occurs within the family group.

   2. Problems associated with individuation include:
      a. Enmeshment: overinvolvement of family members, interfering with individuation
      b. Disengagement: underinvolvement of family members, leading to estrangement of individuated members
   3. Projection of family problems or expectations onto individual members includes:
      a. Scapegoating: One member is blamed or made to suffer for problems in the family.
      b. Identified patient: One member develops more outward symptoms of pathology as a result of family problems.
      c. Labeling: Members are identified by one or more characteristics (e.g., "good" one, "bad" one, "cheerful" one).
      d. Schismatic situation: Schism exists in the couple's relationship, creating a situation wherein the child or children must "take sides."
      e. Skewed situation: Skew exists in the marriage relationship because one member is dysfunctional, leading to an imbalance of roles or wellness in family relations.

II. Functional and dysfunctional families
A. Functional families
   1. A functional family is one that possesses most characteristics of functional families over an extended period.
   2. In a functional family, members effectively shift roles, responsibilities, and interaction during periods of stress.
   3. A functional family may exhibit problematic symptoms during prolonged stress but will rebalance with support to each member.
   4. Specific characteristics of a *functional family* include:
      a. Communicates in a clear direct manner; encourages discussion of issues, even conflictual issues
      b. Has clearly defined boundaries among the family subsystems and clearly but not rigidly defined boundaries delineating the family from the suprasystem
      c. Is flexible
      d. Maintains a balance between change and stability
      e. Develops basic belief patterns that are supported by facts; members are cognizant of their belief patterns and willing to discuss them
      f. Promotes and encourages individual autonomy and growth of members
      g. Resolves problem: clearly defines and names the problem, explores alternative solutions, implements and evaluates the selected solution, and is willing to try another solution if the selected solution didn't work
      h. Defines family members' roles and responsibilities (who does what, when, where, and how)

B. **Dysfunctional families**
   1. A dysfunctional family lacks one or more characteristics of the functional family.
   2. Symptoms arise over time or with stress, during family development, and at life transitions; predisposing factors include:
      a. Marital conflict
      b. Parent–child conflict
      c. Sibling conflict
      d. Acting-out of child (children)
      e. Symptoms in individual (identified patient)
   3. Dysfunction may be transmitted across generations.
   4. In contrast to a functional family, a *dysfunctional family:*
      a. Communicates in a confusing and indirect manner (neither the message nor the target of the communication is clear)
      b. Has unclear and diffuse boundaries delineating family subsystems and either diffuse or rigidly delineated suprasystem boundaries
      c. Is inflexible
      d. Is resistant to change
      e. Develops belief patterns based on stereotypes, myths, and biases; members may or may not be cognizant of belief patterns and are unable to accept challenges to belief patterns
      f. Does not encourage or support individual autonomy among members; experiences enmeshment, disengagement, or triangulation
      g. Experiences difficulty in resolving problems; may have trouble defining and naming a problem, exploring alternative solutions, and implementing a solution
      h. Has unclear definitions of family members' roles and responsibilities

III. Nursing process in family therapy
A. Assessment
   1. Compile a genogram—an informative three-generational map or diagram of family (Fig. 14–1).
   2. Obtain a family life chronology.
   3. Identify ethnic and cultural background, beliefs, and practices.
   4. Determine pertinent definition of family.
   5. Determine phase and tasks of family development.
   6. Assess system-related issues, including:
      a. Boundaries, rules
      b. Roles
      c. Power
   7. Explore relationships, including:
      a. System (e.g., couple, parent–child)

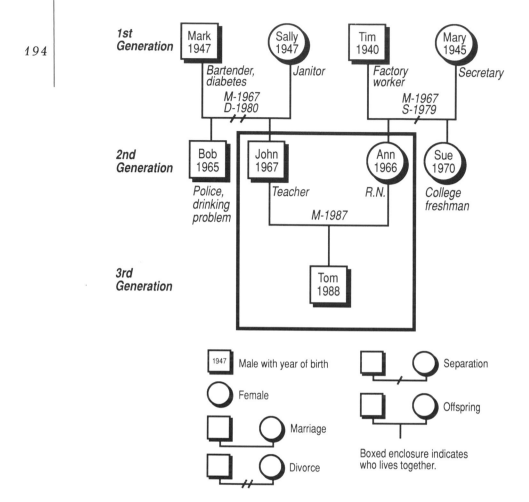

FIGURE 14–1.
Genogram

     b.   Subsystems (e.g., coalitions, triangles)
     c.   Suprasystems—openness to other system impacts
  8.   Assess family communication styles, patterns, and themes.
  9.   Assess individuation of members.
     a.   Identified patient, scapegoating
     b.   Labeling
     c.   Autonomy, enmeshment, disengagement
 10.   Identify problems or symptoms, evaluating:
     a.   Characteristics—whos, whats, wheres, whens, and hows—
         of the symptoms
     b.   Recent changes in family system(s)
     c.   Family's perception of the real problem(s)
     d.   Family's ideas concerning alternatives for solution

B. **Analysis and nursing diagnoses**
   1. The nurse must apply knowledge of systems theory and its relevance to family development and interaction.
   2. Also critical is the nurse's awareness and acceptance of diverse kinds of family systems.
   3. Pertinent North American Nursing Diagnosis Association (NANDA) diagnoses may include:
      a. Ineffective Family Coping
         (1) Related to unclear communication among family members
         (2) Related to sustained marital conflict
      b. Altered Family Processes
         (1) Related to illness of member
         (2) Related to birth of new baby
      c. Altered Role Performance
         (1) Related to confused boundaries within the family subsystem
         (2) Related to unclear delineated family rules, responsibilities, and roles

C. **Planning and implementation**
   1. Be sure to view the family as a system, keeping in mind that no one member of the family has a problem or is the problem (no identified patient); rather, the problem exists within the family and is a family problem.
   2. Be neutral and objective; avoid taking sides.
   3. Focus on the "here and now," the relationships currently existing within the family.
   4. Be observant and aware of nonverbal communication.
   5. Create an atmosphere conducive to therapeutic work.
   6. Be active and direct; stay in control of the session while at the same time being supportive and caring.
   7. Interrupt family members' maladaptive patterns of interacting.
   8. Establish guidelines for communication and for listening.
   9. Model clear communication.
   10. Have family members practice clear communication, maintain eye contact.
   11. Encourage feedback to and from family members.
   12. Give homework assignments to foster communication among family members and provide specific directions for the family's interaction.
   13. Give assignments within the session, providing instruction on how to communicate and allowing family members to practice different communication styles in the session.
   14. Observe and delineate the family's roles, responsibilities, relationships (coalitions, triangles), and behavioral patterns maintaining these relationships.

15. Encourage the development of more efficient boundaries by:
    a. Defining the subsystems existing within the family
    b. Having members of a subsystem sit together, plan activity together, interact together
    c. Encouraging subsystems to listen to information from other subsystems
    d. Allowing and encouraging members to speak for themselves
16. Challenge dysfunctional family behavioral patterns by:
    a. Prescribing the symptoms: instructing the family to continue its behavioral patterns as a means of taking pressure off the family to change (and thus reducing anxiety related to the behavior)
    b. Reframing: rephrasing or redefining the behavior positively to provide the family with another view of the behavior (thus reducing anxiety related to the behavior)

D. Evaluation
1. Family members verbalize awareness of precipitating stressors and of methods to reduce or eliminate them.
2. The family exhibits functional family behaviors (see section II.A).

Bibliography

Janosik, E. H., & Davies, E. L. (1987). *Psychiatric mental health nursing.* Boston: Jones & Bartlett.

Johnson, B. S. (1989). *Psychiatric-mental health nursing: Adaptation and growth* (2nd ed.). Philadelphia: J. B. Lippincott.

Stuart, G. W., & Sundeen, S. J. (1987). *Principles and practice of psychiatric nursing* (3rd ed.). St. Louis: C. V. Mosby.

Wilson, H. S., & Kneisl, C. R. (1988). *Psychiatric nursing* (3rd ed.). Menlo Park, CA: Addison-Wesley.

STUDY QUESTIONS

1. The Samson family reports that they were referred to the clinic by their daughter's teacher, who is concerned because the daughter's grades recently have dropped significantly. When assessing the Samson family, the nurse could infer which of the following data by studying their genogram?
   a. The women in this family manifest the family problem.
   b. Education is strongly valued by the family.
   c. The men are the dominant figures in the family.
   d. The men are better problem-solvers in the family.

2. To better understand the presenting problem, the nurse would want to elicit which of the following assessment information?

   a. a detailed exploration into Mrs. Samson's sister's suicide attempt
   b. a detailed inquiry into Mr. and Mrs. Samson's perception and explanation of their daughter's underachievement
   c. a detailed account of their 2-month-old baby's development
   d. a detailed examination of changes in the marital relationship

3. The nurse viewing this problem from a systems perspective most likely would conclude that the Samson's daughter's academic problems result from:
   a. the child's lack of initiative
   b. the birth of the baby
   c. the mother's depression
   d. mutually reciprocal family interactions

4. Mr. Jones, Mrs. Jones, and Tim, their

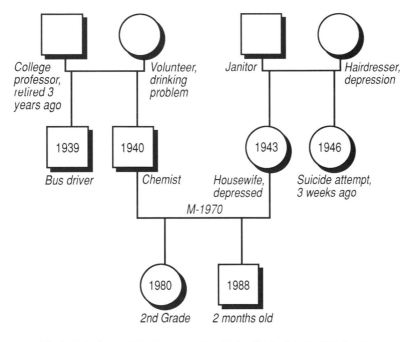

The Smith family reports that they were referred to the clinic by their daughter's teacher. The teacher is concerned because the daughter's grades have dropped significantly. This is the Smith family's genogram.

14-year-old son, arrive at the scheduled time for a family meeting with a family therapist and the nurse. Mr. Jones sits in a chair away from the sofa where Mrs. Jones and Tim are seated. During the session, Mrs. Jones does the talking for Tim as well as for herself; Mr. Jones is quiet and speaks only when asked to reply. Based on these observations, the nurse would identify the relationship existing in this family as a
a. dyadic relationship between Mrs. Jones and Tim
b. dyadic relationship between Mrs. Jones and Mr. Jones
c. dyadic relationship between Mr. Jones and Tim
d. dyadic relationship between Mrs. Jones and the nurse

5. The relationship between Mrs. Jones and Tim would be best characterized as
a. conflictual
b. enmeshed
c. congenial
d. disengaged

6. The nurse observes that the family therapist asks Mr. Jones and Tim to exchange seats. The reason for this is to
a. Reinforce the marital and parental subsystem.
b. Support Tim.
c. Enhance Mr. Jones' self-actualization.
d. Encourage the discussion of spousal concerns.

7. Based on the systems model, which of the following actions would the family therapist likely take next?
a. Encourage Mr. Jones to be more spontaneous.
b. Encourage Tim to speak up.
c. Ask Mrs. Jones to speak for Mr. Jones.
d. Suggest to the family that no one is to speak for other family members.

8. Throughout a family's development, the maintenance of which of the following subsystems most likely would contribute to a functional family?

a. father–son subsystem
b. mother–son subsystem
c. father–mother subsystem
d. husband–wife subsystem

9. When observing the Donaldson family during counseling sessions, the nurse notes that whenever Mr. and Mrs. Donaldson engage in an argument, their 10-year-old son hits his 7-year-old sister, who cries loudly. The Donaldsons then attend to their daughter and reprimand the son, complaining bitterly about their inability to control him. The nurse would identify which of the following dysfunctional characteristics in this interaction?
a. coalition
b. generational conflict
c. triangulation
d. open communication

10. The nurse's most appropriate action in the above situation would be to
a. Recognize that the son is the problem.
b. Support the daughter, who needs protection.
c. Observe the behavioral patterns existing within the family.
d. Sympathize with the parents for having to deal with a problematic son.

11. A family therapist instructs Mr. and Mrs. Donaldson to argue every morning after breakfast and every night after dinner. While they are arguing, the son is to tap his sister on the arm and she is to scream as loud as she can. Which of the following statements best describes this approach?
a. It is not therapeutic because it condones violence.
b. It is therapeutic because it takes pressure off the family to change.
c. It is not therapeutic because it adds stress to the family.
d. It is therapeutic because it promotes insight.

12. In the Peters family, members isolate themselves from the community and

discourage interactions with their neighbors. The family's boundary is
a. closed
b. open
c. flexible
d. durable

13. Which of the following is a characteristic of dysfunctional families?
a. encourages autonomy
b. explores alternative solutions
c. maintains rigid, inflexible roles
d. balances change with stability

ANSWER KEY

1. *Correct response: a*
   The genogram reveals a pattern of depression and suicidal attempt in the females and an absence of symptoms in the males.
   b. Of the eight adults, only two have college degrees.
   c and d. The genogram gives no information about who the dominant figures are or who the problem-solvers are.
   Analysis/Psychosocial/Assessment

2. *Correct response: b*
   It is imperative to understand the presenting problem from the family's perspective. A comprehensive understanding based on the family's frame of reference will aid in developing intervention strategies.
   a, c, and d. Detailed investigation into these other areas would not enhance the nurse's understanding of the presenting problem. It is, however, necessary to discern the family's perception of the impact that these other areas have had on the presenting problem.
   Application/Psychosocial/Planning

3. *Correct response: d*
   This implies a systems interpretation of the presenting problem.
   a, b, and c. These responses imply a cause-and-effect interpretation and not a circular pattern of interactions.
   Application/Psychosocial/Evaluation

4. *Correct response: a*
   The situation describes mother and son forming an alliance that excludes father.
   b, c, and d. The only dyadic relationship described in this situation is the one be-

tween Mrs. Jones and Tim.
Application/Psychosocial/Assessment

5. *Correct response: b*
   Mrs. Jones and Tim's seating arrangement and Mrs. Jones' tendency to speak for Tim are examples of behaviors occurring in enmeshed relationships.
   a, c, and d. There is no overt conflict or congeniality displayed, and the two are not disengaged, underinvolved, or estranged.
   Application/Psychosocial/Analysis (Dx)

6. *Correct response: a*
   This approach taken by the family therapist is designed to challenge old patterns of interacting and to clarify boundaries.
   b, c, and d. Although some or all of these may be enhanced by the therapist's action, none is the primary reason for the action.
   Application/Psychosocial/Implementation

7. *Correct response: d*
   In a continuing effort to clarify boundaries, the therapist would establish rules to promote individuation (i.e., every family member is to speak for himself or herself).
   a and b. These approaches involve individual expectations.
   c. This approach encourages family members to talk for each other.
   Application/Psychosocial/Implementation

8. *Correct response: d*
   Building and maintaining a strong marital subsystem is important in family development.
   a, b, and c. These subsystems are unrelated to the marital subsystem and could be destructive to the marital subsystem.
   Application/Psychosocial/Planning

9. *Correct response: c*

Triangulation occurs when a dyad displaces its conflict onto a third party as a means of reducing tension.

a. The coalition—an apparent alliance between the parents—doesn't capture the dynamics that exist between the parents and the son.

b and d. The conflict is both generational and intergenerational, and there is no indication of open communication.

Analysis/Psychosocial/Analysis (Dx)

10. *Correct response: c*
The nurse's role is to observe the family's behavioral patterns for the purpose of assessment and planning an effective treatment program.

a, b, and d. The nurse should view the problem as a family problem and should be neutral and avoid taking sides (i.e., supporting or sympathizing with one family member).

Application/Psychosocial/Implementation

11. *Correct response: b*
Prescribing the symptoms reduces tension and anxiety and consequently paves the way for the family to make changes.

a and c. This is a therapeutic strategy used to exaggerate the symptoms. When families are given the assignment to act the same, the symptoms lose their intensity.

d. Prescribing the symptoms does not promote insight.

Analysis/Psychosocial/Implementation

12. *Correct response: a*
A system has closed boundaries when the boundaries prohibit the flow of information from the outside.

b, c, and d. The scenario doesn't describe a system with boundaries that encourage feedback (open), that are flexible and adaptive, or that are durable.

Comprehension/Psychosocial/Assessment

13. *Correct response: c*
The dysfunctional family usually has rigid roles and boundaries.

a, b, and d. These characteristics are all common to functional families.

Knowledge/Psychosocial/Assessment

Treatment Modalities:

Psychopharmacology

I. Overview

A. Essential concepts

1. Half-life: amount of time needed for the body to excrete approxi-
    mately half of an ingested drug and the effects to begin to deterio-
    rate or lessen

       2.   Drug interaction: effects of two or more drugs taken together, causing an alteration in the effects of each drug

       3.   Pharmacokinetic drugs: a drug interaction wherein one drug interferes with the processing of the drug in the body, raising or lowering blood levels

       4.   Pharmacodynamic drugs: a drug interaction wherein one drug combines with another to increase or decrease effects

       5.   Tolerance: the gradual decrease of the effects of a drug after continued use of the drug at a certain dosage

B. Nurse's role in psychopharmacology

       1.   Assessment involves:

          a.   Physical examination

          b.   Laboratory studies

          c.   Medication and drug history

          d.   Social and family history

          e.   Mental status examination

       2.   Analysis and diagnosis involve:

          a.   Addressing issues related to side effects and compliance

          b.   Identifying pertinent North American Nursing Diagnosis Association (NANDA) diagnoses (e.g., Constipation, Sleep Pattern Disturbance)

       3.   General aspects of planning and implementation include:

          a.   Keeping current and knowledgeable about drug classification, actions, and side effects

          b.   Maintaining medication administration times, dosages, and so forth to ensure effective blood concentration level

          c.   Monitoring for expected responses and adverse and toxic effects

          d.   Teaching the patient about prescribed medications to promote independence and compliance

          e.   Ensuring patient safety through procedural and preparatory activities (e.g., vital sign and drug blood level monitoring)

          f.   Documenting medication administration and the patient's responses (drug efficacy, side effects)

       4.   Evaluation involves:

          a.   Observing for expected outcomes (e.g., reduced symptoms, elimination or control of side effects)

          b.   Noting the patient's knowledge and compliance levels

C. Patient education

       1.   The nurse must identify the patient's learning needs, problems, diagnoses, and level of understanding before beginning to plan a teaching program.

       2.   The patient's family or significant other should be included in the teaching and learning process.

3. Several issues must be addressed formally or informally during the stabilization period of psychopharmacologic treatment; these include:
    a. Drug name and reasons for administration, including specific target behaviors or symptoms
    b. Administration schedule and route
    c. Expected side effects and a plan for dealing with them
    d. The patient's concerns, feelings, or thoughts about the medication regimen
4. Several issues are of particular relevance to the patient who will be maintained on a psychopharmacologic regimen, including:
    a. Specifics regarding making up missed doses
    b. The need for ongoing monitoring of side effects
    c. Specific side effects that would necessitate immediate notification of the physician
    d. Relevance (if appropriate) of ongoing monitoring of serum drug levels
    e. Drug interactions, including over-the-counter drugs, alcohol, and street drugs
    f. Any applicable dietary restrictions
    g. Sequelae of abrupt medication discontinuation
    h. Side effects and actions that may alleviate specific symptoms
    i. Long-term implications or side effects of medication therapy
5. The nurse can evaluate the patient's comprehension level through the use of a pretest or post-test, verbal summary, or return demonstration.

D. **Patient compliance**
    1. Nursing interventions during medication stabilization include:
        a. Exploring the patient's feelings and thoughts about having to take medication
        b. Monitoring compliance by checking for behaviors or symptoms associated with not taking prescribed medication
        c. Notifying the physician of noncompliance; injectable concentrates or suspension routes of administration may be considered
    2. Increased risk factors associated with noncompliance include:
        a. Lack of therapeutic alliance with the patient
        b. Inadequate patient and family education concerning treatment
        c. Poorly controlled or understood side effects
        d. Polypharmacy
        e. History of noncompliance

        f.   Resumption of the patient's previous life-style or behavior (recidivism)

    3.   Issues that should be addressed to promote compliance include:

        a.   The patient's understanding of the illness and the need for treatment

        b.   The misconception that taking medication is equivalent to being "addicted"

        c.   The possibility of employing a self-medication trial while in the hospital; assessment of capabilities

II. Antipsychotic drugs

A. Indications

1. Antipsychotics are used primarily to treat acute psychotic symptoms of schizophrenia, organic brain syndrome with psychosis, and the manic phase of manic-depressive illness.
2. They also may be used to treat symptoms such as agitation, rage, overreactivity to sensory stimuli, hallucinations, delusions, paranoia, and combativeness.
3. Other indications include treatment of intractable vomiting or vertigo.

B. Mechanisms of action

1. Antipsychotics create a postsynaptic dopamine receptor blockade in the limbic system, hypothalamus, and cerebral cortex.
2. The same dopamine blockade occurs in the basal ganglia, causing extrapyramidal side effects and other undesirable side effects.

C. General considerations

1. Dosage requirements for individual patients are highly variable.
2. Careful dosage titration should be done to target symptom changes.
3. The drug is rapidly absorbed through oral concentrates, suspensions, or intramuscular injection.
4. Serum half-life is approximately 24 hours.
5. The drug accumulates in fatty tissues. When the drug is discontinued, release from fatty tissue continues, and side effects may persist.
6. Antipsychotics have a high therapeutic index and can be given at high dose with minimal risk. Overdose ordinarily is not life-threatening.
7. These drugs are not addicting and do not produce euphoria, and the patient does not develop tolerance to their antipsychotic effects.
8. Effects of antipsychotics on the fetus are inconclusive; use of antipsychotic drugs during pregnancy is not recommended.

D. Selection of an antipsychotic drug

1. The two distinct chemical classes of antipsychotics and their subgroups include:

        a.   Phenothiazines
             (1)   Aliphatics
             (2)   Piperazines
             (3)   Piperadines
        b.   Nonphenothiazines
             (1)   Butyrophenones
             (2)   Dibenzoxazepines
             (3)   Dihydroindolones
             (4)   Diphenyl-butylpiperidines
             (5)   Thioxanthenes

    2.   Low-potency drugs generally produce higher incidences of orthostatic hypotension and sedation but lower episodes of extrapyramidal symptoms (EPS).

    3.   High-potency drugs generally produce higher incidences of EPS, but sedation and hypotensive occurrences are not as common.

    4.   Factors to be considered in choosing a specific drug include:
        a.   Consideration of the patient's tolerance for low- or high-potency side effects
        b.   The patient's positive response to a particular drug in the past, which suggests continued success with the same drug
        c.   Availability of an intramuscular (IM) form of drug for acutely disturbed patients

E. **Administration**

    1.   Small doses of the selected drug are given several times a day.

    2.   The patient must be assessed for tolerance, side effects, and allergic responses.

    3.   The daily dose is increased every 1 to 4 days until symptom improvement is noted.

    4.   Patient response time varies from 2 days to 2 weeks.

    5.   Parenteral high doses may be used initially for more rapid control of agitation.

    6.   Once symptom control is achieved, the daily dosage may be reduced to the lowest effective dose.

    7.   Distribution of the dosage may be rearranged to include less frequent dosings or bedtime administration only.

    8.   If the patient's symptoms are unresponsive after the adequate time (6 weeks), another class of drug may be tried.

F. **Contraindications**

    1.   Antipsychotics are contraindicated in patients with severe central nervous system (CNS) depression due to excessive alcohol, barbiturate, or narcotic use; brain damage; or trauma.

    2.   These drugs also should not be administered to patients with known sensitivity or severe allergic response to one of the antipsychotic drugs.

    3.   Patients with Parkinson's disease may experience an increase in symptoms.

4. Patients with a history of blood dyscrasias are more prone to develop a side effect of dyscrasias than are those with no such history.
5. These drugs should be used cautiously in patients with a history of liver damage or jaundice.
6. Patients with acute narrow-angle glaucoma may experience increased intraocular pressure.
7. Patients with prostatic hypertrophy are at increased risk for urinary hesitancy or retention.

G. **Adverse side effects**
1. Sedation, peaking 2 to 3 hours after administration
   a. Tolerance usually develops within days to several weeks.
   b. Low-potency drugs are more sedative than the high-potency drugs.
   c. A sedative side effect may be advantageous in an agitated patient.
   d. Nursing interventions include discussing with the physician the option of administering a bedtime dose only to avoid daytime sedation.
2. Orthostatic hypotension, generally occurring after 2 to 3 doses
   a. Tolerance develops in several weeks.
   b. Low-potency drugs produce a higher incidence of hypotension than do higher-potency drugs.
   c. Nursing interventions include monitoring orthostatic blood pressure before administering a dose; hold dose if there is a rise in pulse by 30 beats or a drop in blood pressure by 30 mm Hg with a change in position from lying to sitting or sitting to standing.
   d. Instruct the patient to rise slowly and dangle feet while sitting.
   e. If severe, a change to a drug with a lower hypotension profile may be helpful.
3. Seizures: lowers seizure threshold
   a. Patients at risk include those with a preexisting seizure disorder, those taking low-potency drugs, and those withdrawing from alcohol or sedative-hypnotics.
   b. Seizures usually manifest as grand mal type without warning aura.
   c. Anticonvulsants do not protect patients without seizure disorder.
   d. The physician may change to a high-potency drug or decrease the dose.
   e. Nursing interventions include monitoring all patients for seizures and placing patients with a history of seizures on seizure precautions.
4. Depression of hypothalamic functioning

      a.   Signs and symptoms reflect endocrine alterations and include increased appetite, weight gain, amenorrhea, galactorrhea (in women), gynecomastia (in men), and a false-positive pregnancy test.

      b.   Symptoms are more common with low-potency drugs, especially thioridazine.

      c.   Partial tolerance may develop over months or years of therapy.

      d.   The physician may decrease the dose or change to a high-potency drug.

      e.   Nursing interventions include making sure that female patients are not actually pregnant and instructing patients in a dietary and exercise regimen for weight loss.

5.   Anticholinergic side effects

      a.   Symptoms may include blurred vision, constipation, urinary retention or hesitancy, and nasal congestion.

      b.   In geriatric patients, "atropine psychosis" may occur, marked by hyperactivity, agitation, confusion, flushed skin, and sluggishly reactive pupils.

      c.   These effects are more common with low-potency drugs.

      d.   Tolerance develops in days to weeks after initiation of therapy.

      e.   The physician may change the drug to one with a lower anticholinergic profile.

      f.   Nursing interventions include symptomatic treatment such as offering sugarless candy and gum; instructions on a high-fiber diet, fluids, stool softeners, and exercise for constipation; and advice on the avoidance of operating machinery if vision is blurred.

      g.   Treatment for atropine psychosis is IM physostigmine.

6.   Dermatologic effects

      a.   Systemic dermatosis may occur 2 to 8 weeks after treatment; there is a localized rash on face, neck, and chest that usually clears without treatment.

      b.   Contact dermatitis may develop from touching the drug.

      c.   Photosensitivity may result in severe sunburn after unprotected sun exposure.

      d.   The physician may decrease the dosage or change to another drug category.

      e.   Nursing interventions include instructing the patient on using sunscreen and wearing clothing over exposed areas and on immediately washing off with water any concentrate or suspension spilled on the skin.

7.   Hematologic and cardiovascular effects

      a.   Although rare, agranulocytosis may occur within 3 to 8 weeks of treatment.

b. Symptoms occur abruptly and constitute a medical emergency.
c. Symptoms include fever, malaise, ulcerative sore throat, and leukopenia
d. Geriatric females are the higher risk group; monitor white blood cell count.
e. Treatment of agranulocytosis includes immediate discontinuance of drug, reverse isolation, and antibiotics when appropriate.
f. Electrocardiogram (ECG) abnormalities are more common in the low-potency drugs, particularly when combined with tricyclic antidepressants (TCAs).
g. Nursing interventions include monitoring patients with preexisting cardiac disease until baseline and follow-up ECG and vital signs are obtained and evaluated; the physician may change to a high-potency drug.

8. Hepatic effects
a. Rarely, a patient may exhibit jaundice with high fever, abdominal pain, malaise, pruritus, and nausea.
b. Treatment involves discontinuing the drug and providing symptomatic treatment, including maintaining bed rest and a high-protein, high-carbohydrate diet.

9. Neuroleptic malignant syndrome
a. This syndrome is characterized by high fever, muscular rigidity, tachycardia, tremor, hyperkalemia, elevated creatine phosphokinase (CPK), and renal failure.
b. It is a very rare complication; only 50 cases were reported between 1980 and 1985.
c. When it occurs, it does so explosively, with symptoms developing over 1 to 2 days; the mortality rate is 20%.
d. Symptoms may appear at any point in treatment.
e. Persons at risk for this syndrome include those with organic brain syndrome and marked dehydration.
f. Neuroleptic malignant syndrome represents a serious emergency; early symptom recognition is critical.
g. Treatment involves discontinuing all drugs and instituting supportive care.
h. Speculative treatment includes administering dantrolene or bromocriptine.

H. EPS
1. Acute dystonic reactions
a. Symptoms include the rapid onset of severe muscle contractions (usually of the tongue, face, and neck) or extraocular crisis producing torticollis, opisthotonos, and oculogyric crisis.

    b.   The emergence of symptoms often is very dramatic, frightening, and physically painful to patients.

    c.   These reactions account for 10% of all EPS.

    d.   They generally occur within 5 days of treatment.

    e.   Children and young adults are at particular risk for the development of dystonia.

    f.   Males are twice as likely as females to experience dystonia.

    g.   High-potency antipsychotics are more likely to cause dystonia than are the lower-potency drugs.

    h.   Symptoms are readily reversible with prompt administration of one of the antiparkinsonian agents (e.g., benztropine [Cogentin], 1 to 2 mg IV or IM; or diphenhydramine [Benadryl], 25 to 50 mg IV or IM for immediate or rapid action).

    i.   After resolution of the dystonic episode, drug strategies may include changing the antipsychotic drug to one with a lower profile for EPS, lowering the current dose, or administering an antiparkinsonian drug in oral form on a routine basis.

2. Parkinsonian syndrome

    a.   This syndrome is characterized by akinesia (absent or slowed movements) masklike facies, small-stepped gait, cogwheeling and muscle stiffness, bilateral fine tremors, and "pill-rolling" motion of fingers.

    b.   Symptoms commonly occur after 1 to 2 weeks of treatment but may present after several months.

    c.   This syndrome accounts for 40% of all EPS.

    d.   Females and geriatric patients are more likely to experience this syndrome.

    e.   Tolerance does not develop in all patients.

    f.   The dopamine agonist amantadine (Symmetrel) is sometimes helpful; other antiparkinsonian medications may be used as well (benztropine, trihexyphenidyl, biperiden, and diphenhydramine).

3. Akathisia

    a.   This adverse effect is experienced as a subjective restlessness; the patient may be observed pacing, fidgeting, shifting weight from foot to foot.

    b.   The patient may have such complaints as "ants in my pants," "can't be still," or "just have to keep moving."

    c.   Symptoms may be accompanied by leg aches that are relieved by movement.

    d.   Akathisia accounts for 50% of all EPS and is a common reason cited for patient noncompliance with drug therapy.

    e.   High-potency drugs are more likely to cause akathisia than are low-potency drugs.

       f.   Akathisia generally presents weeks to months into treatment.

       g.   Symptoms often are interpreted as agitation and treated with p.r.n. antipsychotics, which can exacerbate symptoms.

       h.   If symptoms are due to agitation, the patient will worsen if the antipsychotic drug dosage is decreased, will improve if the antipsychotic dosage is increased, and will not respond to antiparkinsonian drugs.

       i.   If symptoms are due to akathisia, the patient will generally experience relief from antiparkinsonian drugs or relief if the antipsychotic dose is decreased, and the patient will worsen if the antipsychotic drug is increased.

   4.   Tardive dyskinesia

       a.   Symptoms include bizarre, involuntary, stereotyped, and rhythmic movement of the face and neck; it is characterized by facial grimaces, excessive blinking, frowning, lip smacking or sucking, and tongue thrusting.

       b.   Other findings may include choreiform movements of the limbs and trunk, including pelvic thrusting, shoulder shrugging, foot trapping, and toe movements.

       c.   Tardive dyskinesia is considered a long-term effect of antipsychotic therapy but may occur as early as 4 months after the initiation of antipsychotic therapy.

       d.   Incidence of occurrence ranges from 15% to 50% of all patients receiving antipsychotics.

       e.   Symptoms usually occur after a maintenance dose is discontinued or reduced.

       f.   Symptoms may be masked (but not treated) by reinstituting the medication or switching to another drug.

       g.   There is no known cure for tardive dyskinesia.

       h.   The recommended intervention is to stop all medication and monitor symptoms for remission; however, the physician must weigh the patient's need for antipsychotic medication with the likelihood of relapse.

       i.   Trial drugs such as reserpine and deanol are being used experimentally with equivocal results.

       j.   The Abnormal Involuntary Movement Scale can detect early indications of tardive dyskinesia and should be an ongoing component of treatment.

I. Antiparkinsonian drugs

   1.   Antiparkinsonian drugs include:

       a.   Benztropine (Cogentin)

       b.   Biperiden (Akineton)

       c.   Trihexyphenidyl (Artane)

       d.   Diphenhydramine (Benadryl)

   e.   Amantadine (Symmetrel)
2.   These drugs should not be administered until there is clear evidence of EPS; controversy exists regarding prophylactic use in conjunction with antipsychotic therapy.
3.   Side effects associated with the antiparkinsonian drugs include drowsiness, dry mouth, blurred vision, orthostatic hypotension, weight gain, and photosensitivity.

III. Antidepressant drugs
A.   Indications
1.   These agents are primarily indicated to treat endogenous depression; patients experiencing reactive (exogenous) depression derive little benefit from these drugs.
2.   They are also used in the treatment of anxiety, phobias, enuresis and hyperactivity in children, panic attacks, and chronic pain.

B.   Mechanisms of action
1.   Tricyclic antidepressants (TCAs) block the reuptake of norepinephrine and serotonin at the presynaptic neuron.
2.   Monoamine oxidase inhibitors (MAOIs) inhibit the metabolism of these neurotransmitters, resulting in increased neurotransmitter storage and availability for release.
3.   Both actions reportedly result in a "correction" of the hypothesized neurotransmitters deficit implicated in depression.

C.   General considerations
1.   Accurate diagnosis of depression is critical in predicting and ensuring maximal benefit from these drugs.
2.   DSM-III-R explicates the symptomatology associated with melancholia in depression as including dysphoria, anhedonia, diurnal variation, sleep disturbances, anorexia, and weight loss; the effectiveness of antidepressant therapy is associated largely with the presence of those symptoms.
3.   TCAs and MAOIs are not stimulants, will not produce euphoria, and are nonaddicting.
4.   TCAs are potentially lethal if taken in amounts of 10 to 30 times the daily recommended dose.
5.   Patient response to TCAs and MAOIs may not occur until up to 3 weeks after the first dose.
6.   The TCAs nortriptyline and imipramine have a "therapeutic window" that can be measured in the serum.
7.   Other less commonly used drugs, such as amphetamines and methylphenidate (Ritalin), may be indicated for the treatment of intractable depression.

D.   Selection of an antidepressant drug
1.   The three major classifications of antidepressants are:
   a.   TCAs
   b.   Non-TCAs

c.   MAOIs

2.   Because of the high toxicity of MAOIs, these drugs usually are prescribed only when the TCAs and non-TCAs are not effective.

3.   The choice of antidepressants largely depends on the patient's specific symptoms and behaviors.

4.   The extent of sedative, anticholinergic toxicity, or side effects of the antidepressants is factored into drug selection.

    a.   Doxepin, amitriptyline, and imipramine tend to produce more sedative and anticholinergic effects than do the other TCAs.

    b.   The use of MAOIs tends to be limited to patients who can responsibly adhere to dietary restrictions of foods containing tyramine; failure to do so can precipitate a hypertensive crisis.

5.   Consideration is given to the patient's history of good response to a particular antidepressant.

E.   Administration of antidepressants

1.   In most cases, small doses (25 mg) of a TCA are administered several times a day.

2.   TCA dosage is titrated up by 25% to 50% every other day until a daily dose of 200 to 250 mg is reached.

3.   Serum imipramine and nortriptyline levels can be drawn throughout this stabilization period to track the drug blood level as it approaches the therapeutic range.

4.   After remission of symptoms (lag period ranges from 14 to 21 days), the patient may be placed on a reduced maintenance dose, which should be continued for 6 months to 1 year following an episode of major depression.

5.   Antidepressants should be discontinued gradually. In a change of drug from a TCA to an MAOI, a "drug holiday" should be provided between administration of drugs because of the serious untoward effects that may occur.

F.   Contraindications

1.   With TCA or non-TCA drugs:

    a.   Known cardiovascular disease

    b.   History of seizure disorder

    c.   History of benign prostatic hypertrophy or urinary retention

    d.   Narrow-angle glaucoma

    e.   Active treatment with electroconvulsive therapy (ECT)

    f.   Schizophrenics may experience increased psychotic symptoms if given TCAs

    g.   Elective surgery; should discontinue the drug 1 week before

    2. With MAOI drugs:
        a. Lack of conformance to restrictive diet
        b. Cerebrovascular defects or history of cardiovascular disease
        c. Age over 60
        d. Liver disease

G. **Adverse side effects (TCAs)**
    1. Dry mouth
        a. Nursing interventions include assuring the patient that this is usually temporary; instruct on use of sugarless candies and gums, stringent oral hygiene, and commercial oral lubricants.
    2. Constipation
        a. Nursing interventions include dietary and exercise teaching to include fiber, fruits, bran, and adequate fluid intake; stool softeners or laxatives can be used as necessary.
        b. If constipation is severe, withhold medication and advise physician.
    3. Difficulty voiding
        a. Nursing interventions include monitoring intake and output and checking for abdominal distention.
        b. If severe, withhold medication and advise the physician; catheterization may be needed, and a decrease in antidepressant or the addition of Urecholine may be advised.
    4. Blurred vision
        a. Nursing interventions include advising the patient that this is usually temporary; suggest large-print reading material.
        b. Assess need for eye exam if blurred vision continues beyond one month.
    5. Cardiovascular effects including tachycardia, orthostatic hypotension, and dysrhythmias
        a. Nortriptyline and desipramine have the weakest cardiac effects; trimipramine has the strongest.
    6. Sedation
        a. Effects are usually temporary; tolerance generally occurs within 2 weeks.
        b. Nursing interventions include instructing patient to avoid operation of machinery or driving a car until sedation passes; discuss with physician the option of giving the drug at bedtime in order to avoid daytime sedation.
    7. Anxiety, restlessness, and irritability
        a. Nursing interventions include advising the physician, because a change in drug, dose, or administration schedule may be indicated.
    8. Hypomania
        a. This may mask a bipolar disorder.
        b. Nursing interventions include holding medication and advising physician.

9. Lowering of seizure threshold
    a. Nursing interventions include observing seizure precautions during the initiation of treatment.
    b. Advise the physician if seizure occurs; medication adjustments may be needed.
10. Weight gain
    a. Fluoxetine and trazodone are the least likely to cause weight gain; amitriptyline and doxepin are the most likely.
11. Decreased or increased libido; ejaculatory and erection disturbances
    a. Nursing interventions include notifying the physician, because the medication dose may be changed.
12. Anticholinergic delirium
    a. Symptoms may include agitation, confusion, hallucinations, dilated pupils, tachycardia, and fever.
    b. This is more likely to occur if a TCA is combined with other anticholinergic drugs (such as antipsychotics or antiparkinsonian drugs).
    c. Nursing interventions include promptly recognizing the symptoms and holding the drug; notify physician.
    d. Assist with treatment, which includes IV or IM physostigmine.

H. **Adverse side effects (MAOIs)**
1. In addition to the side effects associated with TCAs, MAOIs may also produce symptoms of diarrhea, abdominal pain, restlessness, insomnia and dizziness.
2. The most serious potential side effect is hypertensive crisis; this occurs when tyramine-containing foods are consumed.
3. Symptoms of hypertensive crisis include generalized headache, nausea, vomiting, pallor, chills, stiff neck, muscle twitching, palpitations, and chest pain.
4. Treatment includes slow administration of phentolamine mesylate (Regitine) and promoting hydration and electrolyte balance.
5. Nursing implications in patient education
    a. Instruction concerning the need to restrict tyramine-containing foods is essential.
    b. Foods high in tyramine are: aged cheese, red wine, beer, yogurt, chocolate, pickled herring, and bananas.
    c. Patient must be cautioned not to continue with over-the-counter products without consulting physician (see section III.I, Drug interactions).
    d. Instruction on the signs and symptoms of untoward side effects, particularly hypertensive crisis, is essential.
    e. Restriction of tyramine-containing foods must occur for 2 weeks after the drug is discontinued.

   I.   **Drug interactions**

       1.   Medications to avoid while taking MAOIs include:
           a.   Cold medications (ephedrine)
           b.   Decongestants
           c.   Narcotics (especially meperidine)
           d.   Local anesthetics with epinephrine
           e.   Weight-reducing or pep pills
       2.   Certain medications should be given in decreased dosages when combined with MAOIs, including:
           a.   Insulin and oral hypoglycemics
           b.   Oral anticoagulants
           c.   Thiazide diuretics
           d.   Anticholinergics
           e.   Muscle relaxants

IV. **Antimanic drugs (lithium carbonate, lithium citrate)**

   A. **Indications for use**

       1.   Primarily used to treat acute manic and hypomanic episodes, and also used in long-term prophylactic treatment of bipolar disorders; particularly effective in the prevention of recurrent manic episodes
       2.   Used experimentally to treat other psychiatric disorders that involve mood disturbance, such as:
           a.   Alcoholism
           b.   Drug abuse
           c.   Premenstrual syndrome
           d.   Pathologic sexuality and phobias

   B. **Mechanisms of action**

       1.   The exact mechanism of action of antimanic drugs is unclear.
       2.   Studies indicate that they interfere with norepinephrine, dopamine, and serotonin metabolism.
       3.   They affect electrolyte balance in the brain and alter sodium transport in nerves and muscle cells.
       4.   It is speculated that lithium corrects an ion exchange abnormality.

   C. **General considerations**

       1.   Lithium is a naturally occurring salt found in minerals, sea water, plants and animals.
       2.   It is readily absorbed after oral administration.
       3.   It competes with sodium for reabsorption in the proximal tubules of the kidney.
       4.   Before receiving lithium therapy, a patient must undergo a complete health history and physical examination, focusing on:
           a.   Renal function: 24-hour creatinine clearance, blood urea nitrogen (BUN), and electrolytes; personal or family history of renal disease, diabetes mellitus; diuretic or analgesic use

        b.   Thyroid function: thyroid blood tests, personal or family history of thyroid disease

5.   Lithium has a success rate of 70% to 80% in the treatment of bipolar disorder.

6.   Lithium can augment the effects of antidepressants and is effective resolving and preventing recurrent major depression.

7.   Carbamazepine (Tegretol) may be used to treat bipolar disorder in patients who are not responsive to lithium or who cannot take the drug.

8.   Valproic acid amide also is used to treat bipolar disorder.

D.   **Administration**

1.   During acute manic episodes, antipsychotic drugs often are used concurrently to manage behavioral and psychotic manifestations.

2.   After psychotic symptoms diminish, the antipsychotic drug dosage can be gradually decreased, then discontinued.

3.   Lithium therapy typically begins with 300 mg t.i.d. for several days, followed by increasing titrated doses until a steady state is obtained.

4.   Typically, a daily dosage of 1500 to 2000 mg/day is required during an acute manic episode.

5.   Lithium has a narrow therapeutic index; the therapeutic dose is only slightly less than the amount producing toxicity.

6.   During lithium stabilization, serum lithium levels are drawn regularly until a therapeutic range is observed.

7.   The therapeutic serum lithium level ranges from 0.6 to 1.4 mEq/L in adults.

8.   The response to lithium is highly variable; the dosage requirement for one patient may be twice the lethal dose in another.

9.   Blood samples for serum lithium levels should be drawn in the morning, 12 hours after the last dose.

10.   Lithium is available in 150-, 300-, and 600-mg capsules; in 300-mg tablets; in 300- and 450-mg time-release tablets; and in an oral liquid form (lithium citrate).

11.   Lithium is rapidly absorbed, with peak effects occurring in 1 to 3 hours; it must be administered in at least two divided doses daily.

12.   After a therapeutic level is reached, it may take up to 1 more week for the patient's symptoms to subside.

13.   Maintenance levels of lithium are generally lower, typically ranging from 900 to 1500 mg/day.

14.   Serum lithium levels should be checked every 2 to 3 months or whenever any behavioral change suggests altered serum level.

E.   **Contraindications**

1.   Elderly or debilitated patients

2.   Thyroid or renal disease

      3. Epilepsy
      4. Severe dehydration or sodium depletion
      5. Brain damage or cardiovascular disease

F. **Adverse side effects**
      1. Nausea, abdominal discomfort, diarrhea, or soft stools
          a. These effects usually are benign and temporary.
          b. Nursing interventions include administering lithium with meals, snacks, or milk or instructing the patient to do so.
          c. If symptoms persist, the dose may be decreased temporarily or another lithium preparation tried.
      2. Tremors, ranging from fine to coarse
          a. Nursing interventions include advising the patient to restrict caffeine products.
          b. The dose may be reduced, given more frequently, or given in a slow-release form.
          c. Inderal may be administered for severe or incapacitating tremors.
      3. Thirst
          a. Nursing interventions include instructing the patient to quench thirst while maintaining a fairly stable fluid intake of six to eight glasses of water daily.
      4. Weight gain
          a. Nursing interventions include obtaining a diet history, advising against fluid and sodium restriction, and encouraging a moderate restriction of calories combined with an exercise regimen.
      5. Muscle weakness and fatigue, usually benign and temporary
          a. The dose may be reduced and given in more frequent divided doses, or a time-release form may be given, lowering the dose and then gradually raising it.
          b. Nursing interventions include assessing rest and activity pattern, protecting the patient from exhaustion by limiting stimuli, promoting safety by discouraging smoking alone, and teaching the patient to avoid operating a motor vehicle while symptoms are experienced.
      6. Hair loss, usually temporary
          a. Nursing interventions include checking thyroid function profile and assessing for hypothyroidism.
          b. If hair loss persists, lithium may need to be discontinued.
      7. Polyuria, usually a benign side effect, but possibly progressing to diabetes insipidus
          a. Urine volume may return to normal with altered dosing schedule, a change in lithium preparation, or use of a time-release form.
          b. Nursing assessment of severe polyuria includes monitoring

intake and output and conducting 24-hour urine collection if ordered.

    c.   Interventions for severe polyuria may include reduced protein and sodium intake; reduced lithium dosage, with a thiazide or a potassium-sparing diuretic; or variations of the above approaches.

G.   Lithium toxicity

    1.   This rare but potentially lethal side effect occurs when ingested lithium cannot be detoxified and excreted by the kidneys.

    2.   Generally, toxicity occurs when serum lithium levels exceed 2.0 mEq/L.

    3.   Signs and symptoms of lithium toxicity include:

        a.   In mild toxicity (serum level about 1.5 mEq/L): slight apathy, lethargy, diminished concentration, mild ataxia and muscle weakness, coarse hand tremors, and slight muscle twitching

        b.   In moderate toxicity (serum level about 1.5 to 2.5 mEq/L): severe diarrhea, nausea and vomiting, mild to moderate ataxia and incoordination, slurred speech, tinnitus, blurred vision, frank muscle twitching, ataxia, and irregular tremor

        c.   In severe toxicity (serum level above 2.5 mEq/L): nystagmus, muscle fasciculations, deep tendon hyperreflexia, visual or tactile hallucinations, oliguria or anuria, severely impaired level of consciousness, grand mal seizure, coma, or death

    4.   Nursing management of lithium toxicity involves:

        a.   Rapidly assess for clinical symptomatology; trust your clinical judgment even if serum level is within or slightly above therapeutic range.

        b.   Hold lithium and notify the physician of assessment findings.

        c.   Monitor vital signs and level of consciousness and be prepared to initiate stabilization procedures if necessary.

        d.   As ordered, obtain serum lithium level, electrolyte and complete blood count (CBC) profiles, BUN and creatinine levels; monitor cardiac status and assist with ECG.

        e.   Assist in further support measures as indicated by the patient's status or as ordered by the physician.

    5.   Nursing implications for patient education include teaching about:

        a.   The generally long-term nature of lithium maintenance therapy; various physiologic and environmental factors that can disrupt the delicately balanced serum level

        b.   Common causes of an increase in lithium level, including decreased sodium intake; fluid and electrolyte loss associated with severe sweating, dehydration, or diarrhea; diuretic therapy; medical illness; and overdose

   c.   The need to maintain a stable dosing schedule (The patient may take a missed dose within 2 hours of the scheduled time; otherwise, he should skip the missed dose and take the next dose at the scheduled time.)

   d.   The need for adequate dietary sodium and fluid intake (six to eight glasses per day) and for replacing fluids and electrolytes during exercise, prolonged heat exposure, or GI illness

   e.   The fact that alcohol may potentiate adverse effects of lithium

   f.   Not discontinuing lithium abruptly but rather tapering dosage

   g.   Not adjusting lithium dosage without consulting the physician

   h.   Not combining lithium with over-the-counter products without consulting the physician (see section IV.H)

   i.   The need for frequent (every 1 to 3 months) serum lithium level evaluation

   j.   Signs and symptoms of lithium toxicity and early indications of bipolar relapse

H.   Drug interactions

   1.   Combining lithium with certain other medications may cause problems; these drugs and the resulting effects include:

      a.   Antipsychotics, which may precipitate neurotoxicity (particularly in elderly patients), marked by EPS, fever, lethargy, and tremors

      b.   Antidepressants, which may increase the risk of manic relapse or shorten cycles

      c.   Aminophylline or theophylline, sodium bicarbonate, and sodium chloride, which may lower serum lithium level

      d.   Diuretics, which cause increased reabsorption of lithium by the kidneys, possibly leading to lithium toxicity

      e.   Tetracycline and spectinomycin, which occasionally raise lithium level and may cause toxicity

      f.   Nonsteroidal antiinflammatory drugs, which may raise lithium level and cause toxicity

      g.   Muscle relaxants and anesthetics, which can prolong neuromuscular blockade of succinylcholine and pancuronium. (Lithium should be discontinued 48 to 72 hours before administration of these agents and resumed when oral intake is adequate after surgery.)

V.   Antianxiety (anxiolytic) and sedative-hypnotic drugs

   A.   Indications

      1.   These drugs are used primarily to treat anxiety and sleep disorders.

2. They also may be used in the clinical management of alcohol and drug withdrawal, as preoperative medications, and as muscle relaxants or anticonvulsant agents.

3. Barbiturates may be used to treat seizure disorders or as preoperative sedatives.

4. Beta blockers may be used to treat stress or specific anxiety resulting in such autonomic symptoms as trembling, palpitations, diaphoresis, and tachycardia.

B. Mechanisms of action

1. Benzodiazepines are thought to potentiate the neurotransmitter gamma aminobutyric acid, producing muscle relaxation.

2. Beta blockers induce a peripheral beta-adrenergic blockade and possibly some CNS effects.

C. General considerations

1. Benzodiazepines, the most widely prescribed drugs in the world, generally are regarded as the drug of choice for treating anxiety and sleep disorders.

2. Benzodiazepines and sedative-hypnotics produce tolerance to their effects within days; cross-tolerance among drugs also may develop.

3. Continued use may lead to emotional and physical dependency; withdrawal symptoms may appear with abrupt discontinuation of therapy.

4. Barbiturates, although inexpensive, have a narrow margin of safety; doses as low as 10 to 15 times the therapeutic dose have proved lethal.

5. Benzodiazepines have a high therapeutic index and are rarely involved in successful suicides.

6. Experts generally recommend that an antianxiety agent and sedative-hypnotic therapy be brief, prescribed for a specific stressor, and used as an adjunct to psychotherapy and other therapeutic modalities in treating anxiety disorders.

D. Selection of an antianxiety or sedative-hypnotic agent

1. The four general categories of these drugs include:

   a. Antianxiety benzodiazepines: alprazolam (Xanax), chlordiazepoxide (Librium), chlorazepate (Tranxene), diazepam (Valium), lorazepam (Ativan), and oxazepam (Serax)

   b. Sedative-hypnotic benzodiazepines (used to treat sleep disturbances): flurazepam (Dalmane), temazepam (Restoril), and triazolam (Halcion)

   c. Non-benzodiazepines (used to treat anxiety and for their sedative-hypnotic actions): meprobamate (Equanil), ethchlorvynol (Placidyl), chloral hydrate (Noctec); antihistamines used to treat anxiety, including diphenhydramine

(Benadryl) and hydroxyzine (Vistaril); and propranolol (Inderal), a beta-adrenergic blocker used selectively to treat anxiety

    d.   Barbiturates: secobarbital (Seconal), pentobarbital (Nembutal), amobarbital (Amytal), butabarbital (Butisol), and others

  2.   Choice of an antianxiety or sedative-hypnotic depends largely on a thorough assessment of the patient's symptoms; a physiologic diagnosis that may present with anxiety as a major symptom must be ruled out.

  3.   Consideration of drug half-life is factored into drug selection.

  4.   Other factors to be considered in choosing a particular drug include:

    a.   The patient's use of alcohol, street drugs, or over-the-counter drugs

    b.   Specificity and quality of the patient's anxiety

    c.   The patient's risk of suicidal behavior

    d.   Presence of specific medical conditions (e.g., liver disease, which would preclude the use of barbiturates)

E. Administration

  1.   Benzodiazepines generally are given orally; an IM form also is available.

  2.   Administration of antianxiety benzodiazepines typically occurs several times daily; specific drug half-life determines dosing frequency.

  3.   Close observation during initial treatment is necessary to assess response and side effects and guide dosage titration.

  4.   All benzodiazepines, regardless of half-life, should be tapered.

  5.   When prescribed to help manage alcohol or drug withdrawal, benzodiazepines may be given in high doses initially, with the patient weaned gradually.

  6.   Sedative-hypnotic benzodiazepines typically are given at bedtime, with a repeat dose possibly given if the patient doesn't fall asleep within a designated period.

  7.   Sedative-hypnotic therapy generally is not effective after 28 consecutive days or so.

F. Contraindications

  1.   Benzodiazepines generally should be avoided in patients with a history of alcohol or drug abuse because of the possibility of cross-tolerance and the increased risk for abuse.

  2.   Patients with uremia or hepatic insufficiency should not be given benzodiazepines or barbiturates.

  3.   Use of anxiolytics or sedatives in pregnant or lactating women is not recommended.

  4.   Inderal is contraindicated in patients with certain cardiac and pulmonary diseases.

G. **Adverse side effects**
   1.   Antianxiety and sedative-hypnotic benzodiazepines may produce side effects associated with CNS depression: daytime drowsiness, ataxia, feelings of detachment, dizziness, and increased irritability. Nursing interventions include monitoring activity carefully to prevent falls, discouraging isolation, and encouraging involvement in activities that may reduce drowsiness.
   2.   Other side effects that may occur with long-term benzodiazepine use include tolerance to effects, dependency, rebound insomnia, and anxiety.
   3.   Benzodiazepine withdrawal syndrome may result from abrupt discontinuation of therapy; it may manifest with tremulousness, insomnia, headaches, tinnitus, anorexia, and vertigo. Treatment involves reinstituting drug administration and tapering the dosage slowly.
   4.   Side effects associated with barbiturates include REM suppression, daytime drowsiness, and a "hangover" effect the next morning.
   5.   Chloral hydrate, in particular, may cause GI distress.
   6.   Inderal may cause insomnia, hallucinations, impaired metabolism of other drugs, lethargy or depression, GI distress, and skin rash.
   7.   Antihistamines may produce sedation, anticholinergic side effects, and decreased seizure threshold.
   8.   Nursing implications in patient education include:
      a.   Explaining that care is directed at providing maximum symptom relief with minimum drug dosages
      b.   Explaining that p.r.n. use of antianxiety drugs generally does not reduce anxiety, because steady drug blood levels are necessary for optimal effects
      c.   Teaching that antianxiety and sedative-hypnotic drugs do not treat the cause of anxiety or sleeplessness, but rather treat only the symptoms
      d.   Cautioning against combining these drugs with alcohol or other CNS depressants because of additive effects
      e.   Cautioning against operating motor vehicles and machinery if muscular coordination is impaired secondary to drug therapy
      f.   Apprising the patient of the side effects and risks of dependency and tolerance

H. **Drug interactions**
   1.   Effectiveness of the benzodiazepines is diminished when combined with excessive intake of caffeine or heavy tobacco smoking.
   2.   Benzodiazepines potentiate the CNS effects of alcohol, barbiturates, narcotics, sedatives, and TCAs.
   3.   Combining benzodiazepines with phenytoin (Dilantin) may enhance toxic effects.

4. Increased metabolism of the following drugs may occur when combined with barbiturates: coumarin derivatives, MAOIs, TCAs, phenothiazines, phenytoin, oral contraceptives, griseofulvin, and rifampicin.

Bibliography

Janosik, E. H., & Davies, E. L. (1987). *Psychiatric mental health nursing.* Boston: Jones & Bartlett.

Johnson, B. S. (1989). *Psychiatric-mental health nursing: Adaptation and growth* (2nd ed.). Philadelphia: J. B. Lippincott.

Johnson, G., & Hannah, K. (1987). *Pharmacology and the nursing process* (2nd ed.). Philadelphia: W. B. Saunders.

Rodman, M., & Karch, A. (1985). *Pharmacology and drug therapy in nursing* (3rd ed.). Philadelphia: J. B. Lippincott.

Stuart, G. W., & Sundeen, S. J. (1987). *Principles and practice of psychiatric nursing* (3rd ed.). St. Louis: C. V. Mosby.

Wilson, H. S., & Kneisl, C. R. (1988). *Psychiatric nursing* (3rd ed.). Menlo Park, CA: Addison-Wesley.

STUDY QUESTIONS

1. An adolescent boy is being assessed for a major affective disorder. All things being equal, if antidepressants are determined to be the drug of choice, which agent most likely will be considered, and why?
   a. carbamazepine (Tegretol), the drug of choice for depressed adolescents
   b. doxepin (Sinequan), generally the first-line treatment for depression
   c. methylphenidate (Ritalin), to promote a sense of well-being
   d. Phenelzine sulfate (Nardil), which produces few side effects and is more rapidly effective than TCAs

2. Ms. Johnson, aged 22, has been diagnosed with bipolar illness and has been taking lithium for over 3 weeks. When returning from a pass to the beach on a warm July afternoon, she complains of apathy, vague GI symptoms, and decreased attention span. What further data would the nurse need to collect in order to accurately assess Ms. Johnson's present symptoms?
   a. the last time she ate
   b. the presence of hypomanic symptoms
   c. her fluid intake while on pass
   d. how she feels about her symptoms

3. The nurse is working with Mr. Leonard, a paranoid schizophrenic, in an effort to improve his compliance with his antipsychotic medication regimen. Which of the following issues should the nurse explore further with Leonard?
   a. the nurse's frustrations concerning his unwillingness to cooperate
   b. the meaning Leonard attaches to having to take medication
   c. whether or not Leonard really needs to take this medication
   d. the possibility that Leonard may need to be reinstitutionalized

4. Which of the following vital sign readings would cause the nurse to consult with the physician about changing a patient's scheduled morning dose of haloperidol (Haldol)?

   a. blood pressure (BP) 124/84, P 92 (supine); BP 126/90, P 84 (standing)
   b. BP 112/62, P 84 (supine); BP 114/80, P 78 (standing)
   c. BP 122/70, P 80 (supine); BP 90/60, P 112 (standing)
   d. BP 130/80, P 100 (supine); BP 120/68, P 110 (standing)

5. Mr. Jones, a client on the nurse's psychiatric unit, is planning on spending several hours at the zoo this Sunday. Knowing that Mr. Jones is taking Haldol 5 mg P.O. t.i.d., the nurse should offer which of the following instructions concerning his pass plans?
   a. Cancel his plans.
   b. Wear plenty of sunscreen.
   c. Restrict his fluid intake.
   d. Drink plenty of coffee.

6. Why is it important to monitor blood pressure in patients receiving antipsychotic drugs?
   a. Orthostatic hypotension is a common side effect.
   b. Most antipsychotic drugs cause elevated blood pressure.
   c. This provides additional support for the patient.
   d. It will indicate the need to institute antiparkinsonian drugs.

7. Isocarboxazid (Marplan), an MAOI antidepressant, has been prescribed for Mrs. Govoni, who suffers from major depression. During a follow-up visit, Mr. Govoni states that it has been 1 week since his wife was first given the medication, and she does not seem to show much improvement. Which of the following principles would be the basis for the nurse's explanation?
   a. MAOIs are long-acting drugs and may take several weeks to take full effect initially.
   b. Mrs. Govoni may need other supplemental drug therapy to make the antidepressant more effective.

c. Mrs. Govoni has been severely depressed for a prolonged period and it will take time for her to respond.
d. Antidepressants act more effectively when one's physical condition is improved.

8. When monitoring a patient who has been recently started on isocarboxazid (Marplan), the nurse would need to evaluate compliance with
   a. submitting to regular laboratory tests
   b. adequate fluid intake
   c. the treatment plan for depression
   d. dietary restriction of tyramine

9. Ms. Trammell has been taking tranylcypromine sulfate (Parnate) for 1 month. One day, she returns from pass with alcohol on her breath. What would be the unit charge nurse's major concern at this point?
   a. that Ms. Trammell may be becoming depressed again and using alcohol to cope
   b. whether Ms. Trammell drank red wine, which could precipitate a hypertensive crisis
   c. that Ms. Trammell's behavior may be disruptive to the milieu on the unit
   d. that Ms. Trammell's behavior suggests noncompliance with her medication regimen

10. Which of the following drug classes share common side effects?
    a. antipsychotics and lithium
    b. antidepressants and antipsychotics
    c. lithium and sedative-hypnotics
    d. MAOIs and lithium

11. Which of the following combinations of drugs would the nurse expect to be given to a patient undergoing ECT?
    a. methohexital and succinylcholine
    b. anectine and butabarbital
    c. succinylcholine and secobarbital
    d. oxazepam and Anectine

12. Which of the following nursing interventions would be appropriate immediately following an ECT treatment?

a. monitoring for further grand mal seizures
b. assessing vital signs and reorienting the patient
c. initiating restraints to prevent injury
d. administering previously held medications

13. For a patient admitted to the hospital with complaints of anxiety, the physician orders alprazolam (Xanax) every 4 hours p.r.n. Several days after admission, the patient approaches the nurse for a dose. The nurse's *first* nursing intervention would be to
    a. Administer the Xanax and evaluate the patient's response.
    b. Explore alternative methods of dealing with anxiety with the patient.
    c. Suggest that the patient discuss the prescribed medication regimen with the physician.
    d. Explain that alprazolam is potentially addicting and discourage its continued use.

14. The nurse should teach a patient that, when taking oxazepam (Serax), to avoid excessive intake of
    a. ibuprofen
    b. cheese
    c. shellfish
    d. coffee

15. For which of the following patients would the use of benzodiazepines be contraindicated?
    a. Joanne, an active alcoholic
    b. Marion, with a history of cholecystitis
    c. Franklin, who just sustained a myocardial infarction
    d. Terri, who suffers from anorexia nervosa

16. Which of the following principles should the nurse keep in mind when planning care for patients receiving antianxiety drugs?
    a. Orthostatic hypertension my occur.
    b. Increased mental alertness may be expected.
    c. Other CNS depressants will potentiate the drugs' sedative action.

d. Enhanced psychomotor coordination is expected.

17. Ms. Richards has been receiving lithium for the past 2 weeks for the treatment of bipolar illness. When planning patient teaching, the nurse understands that it is important for Ms. Richards to know that
   a. She must maintain a low-sodium diet.
   b. She must take a diuretic with lithium.
   c. She must come in for evaluation of serum lithium levels every 1 to 3 months.

d. She must make up a missed dose regardless of the time elapsed since the scheduled dose.

18. Early signs of lithium toxicity include
   a. torticollis
   b. tinnitus
   c. akathisia
   d. diarrhea

19. Patients taking lithium must be particularly sure to maintain adequate intake of
   a. protein
   b. sodium
   c. vitamin K
   d. multivitamins

ANSWER KEY

1. *Correct response: b*
   TCAs are generally considered the first-line treatment for depression.
   a. Carbamazepine is not an antidepressant; rather, it is used to treat bipolar illness.
   c. Methylphenidate generally is reserved for patients with intractable depression.
   d. Phenelzine generally is not administered to adolescents because of the need to restrict tyramine-containing foods.
   Analysis/Physiologic/Assessment

2. *Correct response: c*
   The nurse would suspect that Ms. Johnson is dehydrated; decreased fluid intake or increased diaphoresis would result in a rise in her lithium level.
   a. There is no relationship between frequency of food intake and fluctuating lithium levels.
   b. There are no data presented to suggest hypomania.
   d. This is not relevant to the nurse's immediate assessment.
   Analysis/Physiologic/Assessment

3. *Correct response: b*
   It is important to explore this issue because patients' misconceptions about the need for drug therapy may lead to noncompliance.
   a. The nurse does not need to explore this issue with the patient.
   c. The assumption is made that the treatment of choice for schizophrenia is antipsychotic medication.
   d. This would be a last resort; efforts should be directed toward promoting compliance in the community setting.
   Application/Psychosocial/Evaluation

4. *Correct response: c*
   A rise in pulse rate by 30 beats per minute or a drop in blood pressure of 30 mm Hg when changing position from lying to sitting or sitting to standing is considered indicative of orthostatic hypotension.
   a, b, and d. These values do not indicate orthostatic hypotension.
   Application/Physiologic/Implementation

5. *Correct response: b*
   Photosensitivity may result in severe sunburn in patients taking antipsychotic drugs.
   a. Canceling plans is not necessary; sunscreen will protect against sunburn.
   c and d. Neither fluid intake nor coffee intake has relevance to the nurse's instructions concerning the side effects of Haldol.
   Application/Safe care/Implementation

6. *Correct response: a*
   Orthostatic hypotension is relatively common, particularly during the first few weeks of treatment.
   b. The opposite is true generally.
   c. This has no relevance to the rationale for taking patients' blood pressure.
   d. The need for antiparkinsonian drugs is indicated because of the presence of other adverse side effects such as akathisia or other EPS symptoms.
   Comprehension/Physiologic/Analysis (Dx)

7. *Correct response: a*
   Response to antidepressant medications usually does not occur until up to 3 weeks following initiation of therapy.
   b. The antidepressants do not require supplemental drugs to ensure effectiveness of therapy.
   c. Response to antidepressants usually takes up to 3 weeks, regardless of the severity of depression,
   d. This has no bearing on the effectiveness of and response time to the antidepressants.
   Comprehension/Health promotion/ Implementation

8. *Correct response: d*
Consumption of foods containing tyramine can result in a hypertensive crisis.
- **a.** This is not necessary when taking MAOIs.
- **b.** Although this is a healthy practice, it is not crucial to the effectiveness of MAOIs.
- **c.** Although this is an important issue, it is of critical importance that the patient's diet be monitored during this time so as not to compromise treatment or precipitate a hypertensive crisis.

Analysis/Safe care/Evaluation

9. *Correct response: b*
Red wine, in particular, contains tyramine and, as such, when combined with Parnate could precipitate a hypertensive crisis.
- **a.** There are no data to confirm or discount this at this point.
- **c.** There are insufficient data on which to base this conclusion.
- **d.** This may be an issue, but it is not the nurse's major concern when assessing this patient.

Analysis/Safe care/Analysis (Dx)

10. *Correct response: b*
This is largely due to these drugs' anticholinergic action.
- **a, c, and d.** Few common side effects are shared by these major classifications of drugs.

Analysis/Physiologic/NA

11. *Correct response: a*
Methohexital is a short-acting barbiturate that provides sedation during the treatment; succinylcholine is a potent muscle relaxant given to prevent injury from the seizure.
- **b, c, and d.** Anectine may be given, but butabarbital (Butisol), secobarbital (Seconal), and oxazepam (Serax) are inappropriate sedative-hypnotics and would not be used for an ECT treatment.

Comprehension/Physiologic/Implementation

12. *Correct response: b*
This is the appropriate role of the nurse when caring for patients recovering from ECT.
- **a.** Grand mal seizures are limited to the actual treatment and do not occur in the recovery period.
- **c.** Restraints are not routinely indicated unless the patient becomes agitated; this generally doesn't occur immediately after initiation of treatment.
- **d.** Medications would not be administered until the patient has regained consciousness and awareness of his surroundings; this generally doesn't occur until about an hour after treatment.

Comprehension/Safe care/Implementation

13. *Correct response: b*
In order for benzodiazepines to be most effective, a steady-state serum level must be maintained; use of Xanax p.r.n. would not afford this optimal response.
- **a.** This would not be the nurse's first intervention; it would be appropriate only after alternative mechanisms to decrease anxiety had failed.
- **c.** This intervention does not address the immediate presenting problem.
- **d.** This would be an inappropriate and nontherapeutic intervention; it exudes judgmentalism and overreactivity.

Application/Psychosocial/Implementation

14. *Correct response: d*
The effectiveness of benzodiazepines is diminished when they are combined with excessive intake of caffeine or tobacco.
- **a, b, and c.** No known adverse interactions with these substances have been reported.

Knowledge/Health promotion/ Implementation

15. *Correct response: a*
Alcohol will potentiate the action of benzodiazepines; abuse may occur as a

result of the cross-tolerance between these drugs.

b, c, and d. There is no evidence to suggest that benzodiazepines are contraindicated in patients with cholecystitis, myocardial infarction, or anorexia nervosa.

Analysis/Physiologic/Analysis (Dx)

16. *Correct response: c*

CNS depressants such as alcohol potentiate the action of sedative-hypnotics and antianxiety drugs.

a. This simply does not occur with this classification of drugs.

b. The converse would be true.

d. The converse would occur.

Application/Physiologic/Planning

17. *Correct response: c*

Because lithium is a potentially dangerous and toxic medication, serum levels must be evaluated regularly to ensure maintenance of levels within the therapeutic range.

a. A low-sodium diet would cause an increased lithium level.

b. Diuretic use would result in a decreased lithium level, which is not a desirable effect.

d. Because of the potential toxicity of lithium, missed doses should not be made up if occurring later than 2 hours after the scheduled dosage time.

Comprehension/Health promotion/Planning

18. *Correct response: d*

GI manifestations usually are the initial symptoms of lithium toxicity.

a. Torticollis is a dystonic reaction seen only with the antipsychotic drugs.

b. Tinnitus is a symptom of moderate toxicity.

c. Akathisia is also an extrapyramidal side effect seen with antipsychotic medications.

Comprehension/Safe care/Assessment

19. *Correct response: b*

Because lithium competes with sodium in the distal tubules of the kidney, a fluctuating sodium level results in a fluctuating lithium level. Therefore, "normal" intake of sodium is necessary.

a. Variances in protein intake have no bearing on lithium level.

c. This has no relevance to the maintenance of a stable lithium level.

d. The patient taking lithium has the same need for multivitamins as does a person not taking lithium.

Application/Health promotion/ Implementation

COMPREHENSIVE TEST—QUESTIONS

1. A nurse and patient are talking comfortably about the patient's progress and how he feels about the therapeutic relationship. This is typical of which phase in the therapeutic relationship?
   a. preinteraction
   b. orientation
   c. working
   d. termination

2. The patient talks about a difficulty in his life similar to one the nurse is also experiencing. Feeling upset about her own situation, the nurse suggests that the patient listen to her problem and that they try to help each other. Which interpretation of this situation is most accurate?
   a. The nurse's action is appropriate because sharing things about herself makes her more human to the patient.
   b. The nurse's action is appropriate because she is self-disclosing in a way that could be helpful to the patient.
   c. The nurse's action is inappropriate because self-disclosure is not considered therapeutic.
   d. The nurse's action is inappropriate because the self-disclosure is focused on her needs instead of on the patient's.

3. The nurse says to the patient, "I'm here to help you." The patient says, "I don't want to talk," and turns his back on the nurse. Based on knowledge about the structural model of communication, which of the following statements about this situation is correct?
   a. No feedback loop exists because the patient did not respond.
   b. The patient's verbal and nonverbal behavior constitutes a feedback loop.
   c. The nurse's message is the feedback loop.

d. A feedback loop is not illustrated in this situation.

4. A patient and nurse are in the working phase of the therapeutic relationship. They have been working on how the patient relates to others on the unit as well as focusing on difficulties between himself and the nurse. On the nurse's day off, the patient arranges to get himself transferred to another unit. Which explanation of the patient's action is most likely?
   a. The patient is testing the therapeutic relationship.
   b. The patient does not like the nurse.
   c. The patient is beginning to take responsibility for himself.
   d. The patient takes an appropriate action to solve the problem.

5. A patient states, "People think I'm no good, you know what I mean?" Which of the following responses by the nurse would be most therapeutic for this patient?
   a. "Well, people don't always mean what they say about you."
   b. "I think you're good. So you see, there's one person who likes you."
   c. "I'm not sure what you mean. Tell me a bit more about that."
   d. "What have you done to create this impression on people?"

6. A patient with depression is scheduled for voluntary admission to an open psychiatric unit. When he arrives, no bed is available. The alternative is to place him temporarily on the high-security locked unit. However, this action violates the patient's right to
   a. privacy
   b. receive treatment in the least restrictive setting
   c. retain his civil rights
   d. communicate with people outside the hospital

7. A nurse on the unit is observed as rou-

Answer sheet provided on page 245.

tinely responding to patients in an auto-
cratic, controlling manner with little
consideration for their dignity and
rights. After many attempts to directly
acknowledge the situation with the
nurse in question, her colleagues plan to
meet with the supervisor to express their
concerns about the nurse's unprofessional manner. The plan to go to the supervisor is:
   a. appropriate, because peer review is a
      professional activity used to main-
      tain quality of care
   b. appropriate, because the nurse is
      probably looking for limits to be set
      on her behavior
   c. inappropriate, because it is up to the
      supervisor to evaluate the nurse
   d. inappropriate, because each nurse is
      responsible only for her or his own
      practice

8. Which theorist views human development not in terms of specific ages but
   rather in terms of a needs hierarchy?
   a. Freud
   b. Sullivan
   c. Maslow
   d. Erikson

9. Nurses study various developmental
   theories in order to better understand
   and assess a patient's developmental
   level. Which of the following statements
   best summarizes the shared view of
   most developmental theorists?
   a. Human development is directional
      and sequential.
   b. Human development consists of
      psychosexual phases.
   c. Human development depends on
      interpersonal relationships.
   d. Human development consists of a
      series of situational crises.

10. The idea that maladaptive behavior is
    learned comes from which theoretic
    framework?
    a. behavioral
    b. educational
    c. psychodynamic
    d. cognitive

11. The concept that all behavior is uncon-
    sciously motivated means that

   a. Behavior arises from internal needs.
   b. Stress motivates behavior.
   c. Thoughts motivate behavior.
   d. Behavior is learned in response to
      stimuli.

12. A psychotic patient is given prescribed
    medications and placed on a behavioral
    modification program. This treatment
    plan is based on which frameworks for
    psychiatric care?
    a. cognitive and behavioral
    b. behavioral and biomedical
    c. biomedical and psychodynamic
    d. psychodynamic and stress adapta-
       tion

13. A particular psychiatric unit has a strong
    behavioral approach to patient care. In
    criticism of the behavioral framework, a
    humanist might state that
    a. Behaviorists intrude too much into
       the person's unconscious motiva-
       tions.
    b. Behaviorists overemphasize anxiety
       and inner conflicts.
    c. Behaviorists ignore emotions, intro-
       spection, and the person's role in
       shaping his life.
    d. Behaviorists operate too experimen-
       tally.

14. A nurse observes that a mother seems
    highly anxious when caring for her in-
    fant. Which theorist would say that the
    mother's anxiety is internalized by the
    infant?
    a. Freud
    b. Sullivan
    c. Maslow
    d. Erikson

15. A patient has taken a leave of absence
    from his job as a result of depression.
    Because of his excellent work history,
    the company for which he works is
    holding his position for him until he re-
    turns. The patient constantly says things
    like, "I'm no good. I can't even work.
    I'm a failure." According to cognitive
    theorists, this patient's negative com-
    ments about himself are an example of
    a. thought processes that maintain the
       depression

b. punitive superego and weak id
c. behavior needing modification
d. projection and reaction formation

16. The Jensons, a young couple, just had their first child and moved into a new home. Shortly afterward, the wife's mother, with whom she was very close, died. Which of the above events would be considered stressors on the Jenson family?
    a. having the first child
    b. moving into a new home
    c. mother's death
    d. having first child, moving into new home, and mother's death

17. Which of the following statements is true about the Jensons at this time?
    a. They may all be at risk for developing physical illness.
    b. The newborn will not be affected by these stressors.
    c. Because the positive events will balance out the negative event, they should not experience stress at this time.
    d. They will automatically be able to cope effectively with these stressors.

18. General adaptation theory (Selye's theory) is used to
    a. Teach patients stress-reduction techniques.
    b. Help patients develop awareness of stressors.
    c. Look at life events that require adaptation.
    d. Explain how the body adapts to stress.

19. Which of the following statements about anxiety is true?
    a. Anxiety usually is pathologic.
    b. Anxiety is directly observable.
    c. Anxiety usually is harmful.
    d. Anxiety is a response to a threat.

20. Mr. Johns is a Vietnam veteran who suffers from nightmares and flashbacks about his war experiences. An applicable nursing diagnosis for Mr. Johns would most likely be Fear, related to
    a. Generalized anxiety disorder

b. Dissociative disorder
c. Post-traumatic stress disorder
d. Conversion disorder

21. A child who is hospitalized following a history of abuse develops another personality that emerges in times of stress. Which of the following explanations best fits this phenomenon?
    a. The child dissociates from the self as a way of coping.
    b. The child develops another personality for companionship.
    c. The child has a poor concentration ability.
    d. The child assumes a complete new permanent identity.

22. Why are personality disorders particularly difficult to treat?
    a. Affected persons commonly function in society and rarely come in contact with therapists.
    b. Affected persons have chronic psychotic states and do not benefit from therapeutic processes.
    c. Affected persons use projection so extensively that they do not gain insight during therapy.
    d. Affected persons resist the therapeutic process because they believe they are perfect.

23. A distinguishing feature of antisocial personality disorder is
    a. attention to detail and order
    b. bizarre mannerisms and thoughts
    c. submissive, dependent behavior
    d. disregard for social and legal norms

24. Mr. Powers has been diagnosed with a paranoid personality disorder. He was fired from his job yesterday because his suspicious, defensive behavior was interfering with his performance and office personnel relations. Today he is angry, hypervigilant, and suspicious of others. He believes people are going to harm him and that he needs to protect himself. A relevant nursing diagnosis to address Mr. Powers' immediate needs could include
    a. Altered Nutrition: Less Than Body Requirements

    b. Disturbance in Self-Concept: Self-Esteem

    c. High Risk for Violence: Directed at Others

    d. Social Isolation

25. Mr. Lane, a patient on the unit, is charming and manipulative. He is especially flattering and flirty today. He pays special attention to one nurse, getting her coffee and holding her chair. Which of the following would be this nurse's best approach to this situation?

    a. Accept Mr. Lane's efforts to practice socially acceptable norms.

    b. Reinforce Mr. Lane's attentions to others rather than self-absorbed behavior.

    c. Ask Mr. Lane directly what he wants from her.

    d. Tell Mr. Lane matter-of-factly that he does not need to flatter to get her attention; explore other ways of relating.

26. Because the patient with a borderline personality disorder often expresses intense emotions, the nurse should plan which of the following?

    a. awareness of and support for her or his own feelings and reactions

    b. group interaction where the patient can ventilate intense feelings to several persons

    c. an isolation room experience where the patient can express his intense feelings without harm to others

    d. to ignore the patient's intense emotions and deal only with the content expressed

27. Evaluation is especially difficult in patients with personality disorders for which of the following reasons?

    a. Patients are often withdrawn even after therapy and may not share results openly.

    b. Little change in behavior may be seen over time.

    c. Nurses have personality disorders of their own and may overidentify with these patients.

    d. Patients improve rapidly and wish to move on with their lives rather than focus on improvements made.

28. Evaluation of patients with antisocial personality disorder is very difficult. However, one outcome measure could be which of the following?

    a. increased impulse control and ability to delay gratification

    b. statements of self-satisfaction and good self-esteem

    c. charming, attentive behavior directed to others rather than egocentric focus

    d. statement of realization that many variables are responsible for one's behavior and problems; guilt is not healthy

29. Ms. Smith, aged 30, was admitted to the hospital with a diagnosis of major depression. The nurse would expect that Ms. Smith's symptoms would include

    a. euphoria, loudness, passive-aggressive behavior

    b. social isolation, inflated self-esteem, multiple complaints

    c. insomnia, irritability, grandiose delusions

    d. slow speech, indecisiveness, anhedonia

30. The nurse observes that Ms. Smith stays in bed with the lights off. From this, the nurse would most logically conclude that Ms. Smith

    a. likes her privacy

    b. is socially withdrawn

    c. needs rest

    d. will snap out of it

31. Which of the following would be the best initial nursing intervention for Ms. Smith's withdrawn behavior?

    a. Tell her that she must get out of bed because that's the ward policy.

    b. Spend brief periods of time with her throughout the day.

    c. Approach her in a cheerful mood to enhance conversation.

    d. Reassure her that everything will be okay.

32. Ms. Smith, speaking softly and slowly, reports to the nurse, "Everyone would be better off if I wasn't alive." Based on this statement, the most appropriate nursing diagnosis would be
  a. Ineffective Individual Coping
  b. Social Isolation
  c. High Risk for Violence: Self-directed
  d. Altered Thought Processes

33. Which of the following would be the nurse's best first response to Ms. Smith's statement?
  a. "Nonsense, you're a great asset to your family."
  b. "Why would you think that?"
  c. "Oh, things can't be that bad."
  d. "It seems that things have gotten pretty bad."

34. Ms. Davis, aged 25, was brought to the hospital exhibiting manic behavior. She flirts with males on the unit and wears excessive make-up as well as provocative clothes. The most appropriate statement by the nurse to Ms. Davis would be
  a. "Ms. Davis, you are not acting like a lady. Get control of yourself."
  b. "Ms. Davis, your family would not approve of this behavior."
  c. "Ms. Davis, let's look through your things to find something that would go better with this setting."
  d. "Ms. Davis, you really look great today. What's the special occasion?"

35. After being told that he has terminal cancer, Mr. Gordon gave away his grand piano, which he has always loved. Based on this action, the nurse may conclude that Mr. Gordon is at high risk for
  a. Depression
  b. Suicidal behavior
  c. Grief
  d. Separation anxiety

36. The nurse's discharge plans for a patient who has a diagnosis of depression should include
  a. discussion of outpatient treatment
  b. discussion of inpatient treatment
  c. discussion of the inpatient facilities
  d. discussion of the patient population

37. Catatonic schizophrenia is mainly characterized by
  a. systematized delusions
  b. marked psychomotor disturbances
  c. disorganized behavior and incoherence
  d. auditory hallucinations

38. Which of the following statements best summarizes what is known about the cause of schizophrenia?
  a. The disorder is thought to be caused by disturbed family relations and communication patterns.
  b. The disorder is thought to be caused by brain alterations in the frontal lobe.
  c. The disorder is thought to be caused by a combination of biologic and psychosocial factors.
  d. The disorder is thought to be caused by altered dopamine transmission within the brain.

39. Ms. Enden, a 40-year-old divorcee, holds a full-time secretarial job and functions well at work. Even though her boss maintains an impersonal, business-like relationship with her, Ms. Enden believes he is in love with her. When asked how she knows this, she says it is because they share their love on an "extrasensory level." Based on these assessment data, which psychiatric diagnosis would be most likely?
  a. paranoid schizophrenia
  b. paranoid delusional disorder
  c. disorganized schizophrenia
  d. agoraphobia

40. When formulating a nursing diagnosis, the nurse must differentiate psychotic responses. This means the nurse must assess
  a. how the patient experiences and interprets the environment
  b. how many psychotic symptoms the patient has
  c. how the family participates in the patient's care

d. whether or not the patient hears voices

41. For a paranoid patient who distorts the events in his or her daily environment on the unit, which of the following outcome goals would be most important to consider?
   a. The patient will demonstrate a realistic interpretation of milieu events.
   b. The patient will perform daily hygiene and grooming without assistance.
   c. The patient will take prescribed medications without supervision.
   d. The patient will leave the milieu if events become too stimulating.

42. A patient with paranoid schizophrenia often directs brief, hostile verbal outbursts toward the nursing staff. Of the nursing actions below, which one likely would best deal with this problem?
   a. Place the patient in seclusion when these episodes occur.
   b. Administer p.r.n. neuroleptic medications when verbal outbursts occur.
   c. Set limits and provide a structured, predictable environment.
   d. Minimize the outbursts by walking away when they occur.

43. Which of the following activities would be appropriate for the nurse to implement with a severely withdrawn patient?
   a. art activity with a staff member
   b. board game with a small group of patients
   c. team sport in the gym
   d. no activity

44. The patient looks frightened and says, "The unit is wired up to the FBI, and they're taking my thoughts away." Which of the following responses by the nurse would be most therapeutic?
   a. "These thoughts aren't real; they're part of your illness."
   b. "I don't believe this is so, but you seem scared."
   c. "How long have you been thinking this?"

d. "Let me show you that the unit is not wired up."

45. Ms. Petruccio, aged 45, has a history of depressive episodes and now presents with marital and sexual concerns. She has difficulty with sexual arousal and situational preorgasmia. Her nonassertiveness prevents her from expressing her sexual and other needs. She is slightly overweight and diets frequently. She reports that her marital relationship is generally supportive. Which of the following additional information would be *least* important in completing a sexual assessment of Ms. Petruccio?
   a. physical examination
   b. medication and illness evaluation
   c. sex history
   d. work history

46. Given the above information and finding there is no physical problem, which of the following nursing diagnoses likely would be most representative of Ms. Petruccio's current condition?
   a. Altered Sexuality Patterns related to nonassertive expression of her own sexual needs
   b. Sexual Dysfunction (inhibited orgasm) related to poor body image, nonassertiveness, low self-esteem, and depression
   c. Depression related to marital problems
   d. Disturbance in Self-Concept: Body Image related to overweight condition

47. Based on the diagnosis "Altered Sexuality Patterns related to nonassertive expression of her own sexual needs," which of the following goals would be most closely related to the diagnosis and within the ability of a nurse at the intermediate level of intervention?
   a. The patient will verbalize about her pattern of sexual expression toward males.
   b. The patient will experience sexual arousal and orgasm regularly.
   c. The patient will identify one way to

increase sexual arousal to meet her sexual needs.

d. The patient will discuss the effect of her sex education experiences.

48. Patti, a patient with multiple sclerosis, is concerned about maintaining her sexual enjoyment because she has decreased vaginal sensation. In providing nursing care for this patient, which of the following interventions would be most important?

a. Provide information about the effect of multiple sclerosis on sexual functioning.

b. Explore Patti's attitude about oral sex.

c. Give permission to enjoy any non-coercive, mutually agreed-upon sexual activity.

d. Instruct Patti in sensate focus activities.

49. Patricia has met with the nurse for four sessions, during which time they have worked on improving her attitude about her sexuality and increasing assertive behaviors in trying to meet her sexual needs. All of the following indicate an appropriate focus for evaluation of Patricia's progress in this case *except*

a. The patient discusses her sense of sexual well-being.

b. The patient identifies ways she is behaving more assertively in regard to her sexual needs.

c. The patient expresses dissatisfaction with treatment.

d. The patient's husband uses more foreplay.

50. Stuart, aged 15, was admitted to the psychiatric unit after a suicide attempt. He was involved in a sexual relationship with a 19-year-old male who recently ended the relationship. Stuart is depressed over the loss and also has conflicting feelings about being gay. One nurse working with him has a value that same-sex behavior is a sin. This nurse also believes that sexual orientation is determined early in life and is not cho-

sen by the individual. The nurse has a 15-year-old son. In planning care for this patient, which approaches would be most important for this nurse to use?

a. Use the patient's goal of not being gay as the primary basis on which to plan nursing care.

b. Collaborate with health team members in setting goals for patient care.

c. Focus on the patient's need for protection from suicide rather than on his sexual orientation concerns.

d. Explore ways to modify the nurse's own belief that homosexual relationships are sinful.

51. Stephanie's sexual history reveals that she was sexually molested at age 9 by a female friend of the family. The family has no knowledge of this. Stephanie has dated boys over the past year and states she wants to continue. Her fantasies are primarily focused on a close female friend with whom she has had sexual activity. She does not participate in any group within the lesbian subculture. Based on this information, which of the following would be the most significant evaluation criteria?

a. Stephanie will explore her feelings, fantasies, and sexual behaviors in regard to both heterosexual and homosexual experiences.

b. Stephanie will tell her parents about the sexual experience when she was 9.

c. Stephanie will continue to date boys, identify attraction to them, and receive reinforcement from staff and family for this behavior.

d. Stephanie will explore the lesbian subculture, participating in the activities, to gain support and more acceptance of her lesbianism.

52. Mr. Baker, aged 57, was admitted with a tentative diagnosis of cirrhosis of the liver. He initially denied having a drinking problem but later stated that he is drinking more and has experienced blackouts. Mr. Baker says he can stop drinking whenever he wishes but that he drinks only because of his wife's constant nagging. From this information, the nurse could logically conclude that Mr. Baker

   a. is dependent on alcohol

   b. lacks control over his alcohol consumption

   c. abuses alcohol

   d. has developed tolerance

53. In addition to denial, Mr. Baker also is demonstrating

   a. projection

   b. rationalization

   c. sublimation

   d. displacement

54. Mary Davis, a 22-year-old pregnant woman, has abused heroin for the past 3 years. She is unemployed and obtains money by prostitution and stealing. She also shares needles and other drug paraphernalia because she cannot afford her own. What would be the most important initial nursing intervention for this patient?

   a. Counsel Ms. Davis about her lifestyle and needed changes.

   b. Assess her or his own personal attitudes about heroin addiction and prostitution.

   c. Counsel Ms. Davis about the dangers of heroin addiction.

   d. Review literature on substance dependence and its impact on women.

55. If Ms. Davis continues to be dependent on heroin throughout her pregnancy, her baby will be at high risk for

   a. mental retardation

   b. heroin dependence

   c. becoming an adult addict

   d. profound psychologic disturbance

56. The most common abusive behavior toward a pregnant woman involves

   a. pressure to have an abortion

   b. injury to the abdomen

   c. locking her out of the house

   d. fracture of the tibia

57. Which of the following statements about nonvictim members of violent families is correct?

   a. They do not require intervention because they are not involved.

   b. They often experience more trauma than do actual victims.

   c. They should be encouraged to seek alternative living arrangements.

   d. They commonly experience fear and guilt from their exposure to family violence.

58. The violent family with severe communication problems could best be helped with

   a. individual art therapy for the child victim

   b. one-to-one behavior modification sessions for the abuser

   c. group sessions using a family systems model

   d. long-term marital counseling for the parents

59. A known previous victim of sexual abuse comes for a routine clinic appointment. She complains of burning on urination. The nurse is aware that the patient and her family have been in treatment, and local agencies believe the case is successfully resolved. The patient is reluctant to discuss other symptoms, tells the nurse to "forget it," and seems alarmed at the nurse's interest. Which of the following should the nurse conclude about the patient's unwillingness to discuss the problem?

   a. The patient initially exaggerated the symptom in order to get attention.

   b. Previous sexual abuse is unrelated to the symptom because other treatment providers are satisfied that abuse has stopped.

   c. The nurse should drop the subject to avoid making the patient more uncomfortable.

   d. The nurse needs more information to assess the patient's health care needs.

60. In assessing whether the patient can remain safely in the home, the nurse must consider all of the following factors *except*

240

a. the availability of acceptable community shelters
b. the ability of the nonabusing caretaker to intervene on the patient's behalf
c. the patient's possible response to relocation of the abuser only
d. the family's socioeconomic status

61. Psychodynamic theory stresses the importance of which of the following factors in understanding sexual abuse?
a. personal history of abuse for abuser, diminished ego strength
b. observation of incest in childhood, poor models of appropriate family role behavior
c. overcoming internal controls to abuse, overriding external inhibitions to abuse
d. the view that women are subject to male domination, the conviction that children are property

62. Mary, aged 15, was admitted to an inpatient adolescent psychiatric ward because she refuses to eat. Which of the following assessment data would lead to a diagnosis of major depression as opposed to anorexia nervosa?
a. She induces vomiting after meals.
b. She hides food.
c. She says that food no longer tastes good.
d. She prepares elaborate meals.

63. Because Mary is socially isolated, she is assigned to group therapy, which meets for 1½ hours Mondays through Thursdays. Which of the following would be an appropriate short-term goal for group therapy?
a. Mary will introduce a topic for discussion.
b. Mary will summarize the group process.
c. Mary will attend group therapy.
d. Mary will talk in the group.

64. Mary says, "I don't want people to know that I'm in this place." What would be the nurse's best response?
a. "Tell me more about what you're feeling right now."
b. "Tell me why you said that."
c. "Tell me what people you're talking about."
d. "Tell me what you want me to do."

65. A young adolescent girl who appears extremely emaciated is brought to the inpatient unit. After reviewing her medical and psychiatric history, the nurse thinks, "How could her parents let this poor girl deteriorate like this?" At this point, what would be the nurse's best action?
a. Approach this adolescent's parents with this question.
b. Talk to the nursing supervisor about her or his thoughts.
c. Be especially kind to this poor adolescent.
d. Tell the other nurses about these insensitive parents.

66. The nurse's review of this adolescent's records revealed that her name is Susan and that she is 16 years old, does well in school, and is well versed in food preparation. The nurse enjoys hearing Susan talk about different foods and menus. On being told by colleagues that this action is nontherapeutic, the nurse
a. agrees, because the focus of this interaction is on food
b. disagrees, because this interaction provides Susan with a social outlet
c. agrees, because Susan dominates the discussion
d. disagrees, because this interaction enhances Susan's self-confidence

67. Upon discharge, the nurse would expect Susan's
a. socialization skills to increase
b. weight to increase
c. Interest to increase
d. Personal hygiene to improve

68. A 13-year-old patient says, "You are really great. You know the answers to everything." The nurse responds, "Thanks, I do my best." This response is
a. helpful, because it supports the child's beliefs

b. helpful, because it enhances the child's self-esteem

c. not helpful, because it reinforces an unrealistic view of the nurse as all-knowing

d. not helpful, because it reinforces the child's view of the world as good

69. Which of the following therapies is most commonly involved in a milieu therapy setting?
   a. behavior modification therapy
   b. art therapy
   c. play therapy
   d. dance therapy

70. Which three balancing factors are assessed and worked with in the crisis intervention model?
   a. communication patterns, coping skills, problem solving
   b. situational support, expression of feelings, anxiety
   c. perception of event, situational support, coping skills
   d. coping skills, reality testing, cognitive distortions

71. A seriously ill patient dies much sooner than expected. Family members are called in and, when they arrive, are told about the death. At this time, the nurse can expect family members to initially
   a. Share fond memories about the deceased.
   b. Demonstrate shock and disbelief.
   c. Exhibit helplessness and withdrawal.
   d. State how much they miss the deceased person.

72. The person who does not let himself or herself experience sorrow and pain when a loved one dies
   a. may develop depression or illness if grief is not resolved
   b. serves as a healthy role model for others who have experienced loss
   c. will forget the loved one if grief is not experienced
   d. probably is an insensitive person

73. Mrs. Jonas, aged 53, recently lost her husband of 25 years. Although she has always been healthy and recently had a physical examination showing no abnormalities, she now experiences shortness of breath alternated with heavy sighs and complains of weakness. Which of the following statements best describes these symptoms?
   a. They require further assessment by diagnostic testing.
   b. They most likely reflect the early phase of grieving.
   c. They probably are unrelated to her husband's death.
   d. They point to maladaptive grieving.

74. The primary goal of crisis intervention is to
   a. Return the patient to normal functioning.
   b. Develop insight into reasons why a person is crisis-prone.
   c. Change coping skills and behavioral patterns.
   d. Learn to relate better to others.

75. If a crisis remains unresolved for more than 3 months, what might be a more appropriate analysis of the patient's situation?
   a. The patient has not received adequate support.
   b. The patient may be experiencing an adjustment disorder.
   c. The patient is not amenable to crisis intervention.
   d. The patient is not cooperating well with therapy.

76. Two nurses are co leading group therapy for seven chronic psychiatric inpatients. They observe that the group members appear anxious and are looking to them for answers. The group is most likely in which phase of development?
   a. working phase
   b. initiation phase
   c. conflict resolution phase
   d. termination phase

77. During this phase, the primary goal is to
   a. promote self-awareness
   b. provide minimal directions
   c. identify conflicts

d. clarify group purpose

78. One of the nurses says, "This is our group and we meet to learn different ways of talking to people. It is important that we practice listening. Our group is designed to help with talking and listening." This response is
   a. nontherapeutic because it restricts group spontaneity
   b. therapeutic because it enhances cohesiveness
   c. nontherapeutic because it does not address norms
   d. therapeutic because it prevents the development of conflict

79. As the group progresses, the nurses observe that the group members are extremely critical of one member. In order to be effective, these nurses should
   a. Continue observation and document what is happening.
   b. Tell these group members that they are acting-out.
   c. Help the group to recognize and understand what is happening.
   d. Realize that this happens in groups.

80. These nurses will conclude that group therapy is progressing well if group members
   a. begin to comment on their behavior
   b. continue to ask the nurses for advice
   c. find someone outside the group to scapegoat
   d. focus on their past relationships

81. Group members have worked very hard, and the nurses remind them that termination is nearing. Termination would be considered successful if group members
   a. decide to continue
   b. evaluate group progress
   c. focus on their positive experiences
   d. stop attending before termination is effective

82. Two patients in the group always sit next to each other and talk to each other during the session. What would be the nurse's best action in addressing this situation?
   a. Ask them to stop talking to each other.

   b. Ask them to share their conversation with the group.
   c. Ask them to change seats.
   d. Ask them to leave the group.

83. In an inpatient setting for delinquent boys, the nurse observes that the day room is noisy, has poor ventilation, and has chairs in disrepair. The nurse also observes that the boys sit or stand by themselves with minimal verbal exchange and that no staff members are in the day room. These observations constitute the nurse's
   a. assessment of behavior in the milieu
   b. implementation for behavior change in the milieu
   c. evaluation of behavioral change in the milieu
   d. plans for behavioral change in the milieu

84. Mr. Dreger and Mr. Hernandez have lived together for the past 5 years as a homosexual couple. They tell the nurse that their relationship is deteriorating. The nurse should first
   a. Tell them to separate.
   b. Recognize his or her own feelings about homosexuality.
   c. Teach them adaptive ways of dealing with heterosexuals.
   d. Discuss the benefits of discontinuing their relationship.

85. Jane, aged 14, lives with her mother, Mrs. Dan, and her maternal grandmother, Mrs. Thomas. Mrs. Thomas criticizes Mrs. Dan on the discipline of Jane, who talks back, disobeys, and makes bad grades. Mrs. Dan and Jane have their biggest verbal altercation around school work. The public health nurse suggests that Mrs. Dan and Jane spend 1 hour together during the week doing something that both of them enjoy. In this situation, the nurse has
   a. prescribed the symptom
   b. reframed
   c. given a homework assignment
   d. given a within-session assignment

86. The purpose of the nurse's suggestion is to

a. enhance the grandmother's position
b. promote understanding
c. provide Jane with a role model
d. develop new patterns of interacting between Jane and Mrs. Dan

87. On the nurse's next visit, Jane reports that she and her mother did not do anything for fun. The nurse concludes that this intervention was
   a. a failure, because the family didn't comply with the homework assignment
   b. a success, because the family's response provided information about the family's readiness for change
   c. a failure, because the family made no progress
   d. a success, because the family returned for this session

88. The nurse tells the family that Mrs. Thomas's criticisms are a way to help Mrs. Dan develop her disciplinary skills, to help Mrs. Dan become a better mother. This is an example of
   a. prescribing the symptoms
   b. reframing
   c. giving an assignment
   d. emphasizing feelings

89. An appropriate evaluation criterion for the nurse's intervention would be
   a. Mrs. Thomas gives suggestions on child rearing to Mrs. Dan.
   b. Jane tells her grandmother to stop interfering.
   c. Mrs. Dan and Jane have at least one enjoyable experience together.
   d. Mrs. Dan tells Mrs. Thomas to assume the parental responsibilities.

90. An appropriate nursing diagnosis for a family would be
   a. Sensory-Perceptual Alteration: Visual
   b. Impaired Verbal Communication
   c. Disturbance in Self-Concept
   d. Sleep Pattern Disturbance

91. One of the primary tasks of a newlywed couple is to
   a. become economically secure
   b. renegotiate relationships with their families of origin

c. plan for becoming parents
d. provide care for aging parents

92. Mr. Joad, aged 26, has been a patient on the psychiatric unit for 2 weeks. He has a diagnosis of schizophrenia and has recently been started on trifluoperazine (Stelazine) 2 mg P.O. t.i.d. Mr. Joad complains that his neck muscles are painfully stiff and getting more tense as time progresses. Given this data, the nurse would suspect that Mr. Joad is experiencing
   a. tension related to his illness
   b. an acute dystonic reaction
   c. symptoms of pseudoparkinsonism
   d. toxic effects from the antipsychotic medication

93. The nurse's assessment of Mr. Joad's complaints is based largely on knowledge of pharmacologic principles. Which of the following statements about his antipsychotic medication regimen is correct?
   a. High-potency drugs such as trifluoperazine result in higher incidences of such side effects as torticollis.
   b. Antipsychotic drugs commonly produce this reaction, accounting for the routine administration of prophylactic antiparkinsonian drugs.
   c. This particular reaction suggests that the patient probably will not respond favorably to this medication regimen.
   d. High levels of antipsychotic medication often result in toxic side effects during the stabilization period.

94. While developing the plan of care, the nurse takes into consideration that, besides neck pain, Mr. Joad probably is feeling
   a. relaxed
   b. sad
   c. scared
   d. relieved

95. Immediate nursing intervention for Mr. Joad should be directed toward

a. obtaining a blood sample to determine the extent of toxicity
b. suggesting that the physician discontinue the medication
c. administering diphenhydramine (Benadryl) IM
d. teaching relaxation techniques

96. Within one half hour of nursing intervention, Mr. Joad reports that his neck is feeling looser and less painful. Further management of this side effect may be accomplished through all of the following actions *except*
a. administering an antiparkinsonian drug routinely
b. increasing the antipsychotic medication
c. decreasing the antipsychotic medication
d. changing to a low-potency antipsychotic medication

Answer Sheet for Comprehensive Exam

With a pencil, blacken the circle under the option you have chosen for your correct answer.

	A B C D		A B C D		A B C D
1.	○ ○ ○ ○	21.	○ ○ ○ ○	41.	○ ○ ○ ○
2.	○ ○ ○ ○	22.	○ ○ ○ ○	42.	○ ○ ○ ○
3.	○ ○ ○ ○	23.	○ ○ ○ ○	43.	○ ○ ○ ○
4.	○ ○ ○ ○	24.	○ ○ ○ ○	44.	○ ○ ○ ○
5.	○ ○ ○ ○	25.	○ ○ ○ ○	45.	○ ○ ○ ○
6.	○ ○ ○ ○	26.	○ ○ ○ ○	46.	○ ○ ○ ○
7.	○ ○ ○ ○	27.	○ ○ ○ ○	47.	○ ○ ○ ○
8.	○ ○ ○ ○	28.	○ ○ ○ ○	48.	○ ○ ○ ○
9.	○ ○ ○ ○	29.	○ ○ ○ ○	49.	○ ○ ○ ○
10.	○ ○ ○ ○	30.	○ ○ ○ ○	50.	○ ○ ○ ○
11.	○ ○ ○ ○	31.	○ ○ ○ ○	51.	○ ○ ○ ○
12.	○ ○ ○ ○	32.	○ ○ ○ ○	52.	○ ○ ○ ○
13.	○ ○ ○ ○	33.	○ ○ ○ ○	53.	○ ○ ○ ○
14.	○ ○ ○ ○	34.	○ ○ ○ ○	54.	○ ○ ○ ○
15.	○ ○ ○ ○	35.	○ ○ ○ ○	55.	○ ○ ○ ○
16.	○ ○ ○ ○	36.	○ ○ ○ ○	56.	○ ○ ○ ○
17.	○ ○ ○ ○	37.	○ ○ ○ ○	57.	○ ○ ○ ○
18.	○ ○ ○ ○	38.	○ ○ ○ ○	58.	○ ○ ○ ○
19.	○ ○ ○ ○	39.	○ ○ ○ ○	59.	○ ○ ○ ○
20.	○ ○ ○ ○	40.	○ ○ ○ ○	60.	○ ○ ○ ○

Answer Sheet for Comprehensive Exam

	A	B	C	D		A	B	C	D		A	B	C	D
61.	○	○	○	○	73.	○	○	○	○	85.	○	○	○	○
62.	○	○	○	○	74.	○	○	○	○	86.	○	○	○	○
63.	○	○	○	○	75.	○	○	○	○	87.	○	○	○	○
64.	○	○	○	○	76.	○	○	○	○	88.	○	○	○	○
65.	○	○	○	○	77.	○	○	○	○	89.	○	○	○	○
66.	○	○	○	○	78.	○	○	○	○	90.	○	○	○	○
67.	○	○	○	○	79.	○	○	○	○	91.	○	○	○	○
68.	○	○	○	○	80.	○	○	○	○	92.	○	○	○	○
69.	○	○	○	○	81.	○	○	○	○	93.	○	○	○	○
70.	○	○	○	○	82.	○	○	○	○	94.	○	○	○	○
71.	○	○	○	○	83.	○	○	○	○	95.	○	○	○	○
72.	○	○	○	○	84.	○	○	○	○	96.	○	○	○	○

COMPREHENSIVE TEST—ANSWER KEY

1. **Correct response: d**
   Termination is an important phase in the therapeutic relationship, during which the nurse and patient evaluate the patient's progress and goal attainment and explore how the therapeutic relationship was experienced. It is also important to deal with feelings about termination during this phase.
   a, b, and c. These refer to the other phases of the nurse–patient relationship.
   Comprehension/Psychosocial/Implementation

2. **Correct response: d**
   Although self-disclosure can be therapeutic, in this instance the nurse wants to share information about herself out of her own needs and anxiety. When self-disclosure is used, it must be focused on the patient's needs.
   a and b. In this instance, the nurse is looking for help herself.
   c. Self-disclosure can be therapeutic if carefully used.
   Application/Safe care/Implementation

3. **Correct response: b**
   The structural model of communication consists of sender, receiver, message, context, and feedback loop. Feedback refers to the receiver's verbal or behavioral response. In this instance, the feedback response is dysfunctional because the message contained is unclear.
   a and d. The patient's verbal and nonverbal behavior does constitute a response.
   c. The nurse is the sender of the message.
   Comprehension/Psychosocial/Assessment

4. **Correct response: a**
   The patient tests the relationship by acting-out. Instead of exploring with the nurse how he feels about the way they are working together, he precipitously decides to move to a different unit. The patient acted in a way that disrupted the therapeutic relationship.
   b, c, and d. The patient has avoided working out conflicts with both his roommate and the nurse.
   Analysis/Psychosocial/Evaluation

5. **Correct response: c**
   When a patient makes vague, global statements, the therapeutic approach is to seek clarification. Seeking clarification helps the patient become more aware of his thoughts, feelings, and ideas.
   a, b, and d. None of these responses would be therapeutic.
   Application/Psychosocial/Implementation

6. **Correct response: b**
   Placing a patient in a treatment setting with more restrictions than necessary violates the patient's rights.
   a, c, and d. These also are patient rights but are not applicable in this example.
   Comprehension/Safe care/Evaluation

7. **Correct response: a**
   The ANA's Standards of Psychiatric and Mental Health Practice call for peer review as a mechanism for maintaining quality assurance. In the situation described, it would be better if a formal peer review system were in place to evaluate the nurses' performance. However, the nurses are correct in expressing their concerns to the supervisor.
   b, c, and d. These responses do not address the nurses' responsibilities for upholding professional standards of practice.
   Application/Safe care/Evaluation

8. **Correct response: c**
   Maslow views human development as a process of needs fulfillment. Basic physiologic and safety needs must be met before a person can grow toward psycho-

logic and spiritual fulfillment. The highest level of need is self-actualization, achieving autonomy and full functioning.

a, b, and **d.** Freud, Sullivan, and Erikson all view human development in terms of chronologic stages.

Knowledge/Physiologic/Assessment

9. *Correct response: a*
Most developmental theorists use a system of chronologic growth to explain human development. Human development is seen as an orderly process.
   b. This reflects intrapsychic theory.
   c. This refers to Sullivan's approach.
   d. This is not a developmental approach.

Comprehension/Psychosocial/Assessment

10. *Correct response: a*
Behavioral theory views maladaptive behavior as a learned response that is reinforced in the environment.
   b. Education is not a theoretic framework.
   c. The psychodynamic framework views maladaptive behavior as an interpsychic or interpersonal process.
   d. The cognitive framework views maladaptive behavior as the result of faulty thinking patterns.

Comprehension/Psychosocial/Assessment

11. *Correct response: a*
The idea that behavior is motivated and has meaning comes from the psychodynamic framework. According to the psychodynamic perspective, behavior arises from wishes or intentions. Much of what motivates behavior comes from the unconscious.
   b, c, and **d.** These responses do not address the internal forces thought to motivate behavior.

Comprehension/Psychosocial/Assessment

12. *Correct response: b*
This question shows how theoretic frameworks can be combined to give

comprehensive psychiatric care. The biomedical framework views psychiatric conditions as biologic abnormalities. Medications used to control psychotic symptoms alter neurotransmitter activities in the brain. A behavioral modification program is based on the behavioral approach to mental disorder.
   a, c, and **d.** These are other frameworks for care.

Comprehension/Physiologic/Implementation

13. *Correct response: c*
Because behaviorists focus mainly on the behaviors and techniques for modifying them, critics believe that the person's emotional aspects are ignored.
   a and **b.** These are common criticisms of the psychodynamic approach.
   d. Experimentation is actually a strength of the behavioral framework, not a criticism.

Analysis/Psychosocial/Evaluation

14. *Correct response: b*
Sullivan believed that Freud's developmental theory was too focused on intrapsychic processes. Sullivan believed that a child develops a sense of self from the appraisal received from significant others. If the mother has a lot of anxiety, the infant will internalize this into his sense of self.
   a, c, and **d.** These theorists place less focus on interpersonal aspects of development.

Comprehension/Psychosocial/Assessment

15. *Correct response: a*
Even though feedback has been given regarding the valued place this patient has in his job, he persists in thinking he is "a failure." These thoughts will keep him feeling depressed.
   b, c, and **d.** These are not cognitive explanations of depression.

Application/Psychosocial/Assessment

16. *Correct response: d*
Both negative and positive life changes

and developmental events are considered stressful.

a, b, and c. These are correct but incomplete answers.

Knowledge/Psychosocial/Assessment

17. *Correct response: a*

Research shows that both positive and negative events can be stressful, and if these occur in combination, they can render the person more vulnerable to physical illness.

b. The infant can be affected by parental stress.

c and d. These are false statements about stress.

Comprehension/Health promotion/Assessment

18. *Correct response: d*

The body goes through predictable stages no matter what the nature of the stressor. The first stage is alarm reaction, the second resistance, and the third exhaustion if the stress continues.

a, b, and c. The general adaptation theory does not address these aspects of stress.

Knowledge/Physiologic/Assessment

19. *Correct response: d*

Anxiety is a response to a threat that increases alertness and motivation.

a, b, and c. These statements are untrue.

Knowledge/Psychosocial/Assessment

20. *Correct response: c*

Anxiety related to post-traumatic stress disorder develops in response to major traumatic events such as war, rape, attack, or torture. The disorder manifests with periods of acute anxiety, nightmares, and flashbacks in which the person is reexperiencing the traumatic experiences.

a, b, and d. These disorders are not described in the situation.

Knowledge/Psychosocial/Analysis (Dx)

21. *Correct response: a*

By developing a new personality, the

child dissociates from the stress of being abused.

b. In multiple personality, the emerging personality takes full control of the person.

c. The phenomenon of multiple personality represents a coping problem, not a concentration problem.

d. The new personality is not permanent; rather, the person switches between personalities.

Comprehension/Psychosocial/Analysis (Dx)

22. *Correct response: a*

Persons with personality disorders typically function in the mainstream of society.

b. Personality disorder does not involve psychosis.

c. Not all personality disorders involve projection.

d. Affected persons do not often seek treatment.

Comprehension/Health promotion/Planning

23. *Correct response: d*

Disregard for established social and legal norms is a common characteristic of antisocial personality disorder.

a, b, and c. These characteristics occur in obsessive-compulsive, schizoid or schizotypal, and dependent personality disorders, respectively.

Comprehension/Psychosocial/Assessment

24. *Correct response: c*

This patient's angry, suspicious behavior could precipitate "self-protective" behavior harmful to others.

a, b, and d. These diagnoses are not supported by the data and are not very pertinent.

Analysis/Safe care/Analysis (Dx)

25. *Correct response: d*

A matter-of-fact approach and exploration of new ways to relate may assist Mr. Lane to modify his behavior.

a and b. These responses would be inappropriate, because this patient is not sincerely attending to the nurse or others.

   c. This approach would not elicit a sincere answer or facilitate new behavior.

Analysis/Safe care/Implementation

26. *Correct response: a*

Intense emotions are easily communicated to others, including the nurse. Self-awareness and support are important.

   b, c, and d. These factors will not help the patient learn to modify his explosive, intense behavior.

Application/Safe care/Planning

27. *Correct response: b*

Behavioral changes often are subtle in persons with personality disorders.

   a and d. These are incorrect statements.

   c. This statement could be true, but it would not be the reason for the difficult evaluation.

Comprehension/Safe care/Evaluation

28. *Correct response: a*

This outcome indicates change and improvement in behavior patterns typical of antisocial personality disorders.

   b, c, and d. These outcomes do not show change or improvement in antisocial behavior patterns.

Analysis/Safe care/Evaluation

29. *Correct response: d*

All three are symptoms of major depression.

   a, b, and c. Euphoria, inflated self-esteem, and grandiose delusions are characteristic of bipolar disorder.

Comprehension/Psychosocial/Assessment

30. *Correct response: b*

A predominant symptom of major depression is social isolation.

   a, c, and d. Any of these three assumptions would com-

municate disinterest and could further enhance the patient's negative self-esteem.

Comprehension/Psychosocial/Analysis (Dx)

31. *Correct response: b*

Spending brief periods of time with the patient communicates respect, acceptance, and understanding.

   a, c, and d. These approaches would not be appropriate for this situation.

Application/Safe care/Implementation

32. *Correct response: c*

The nurse should always assess for risk of suicide in persons with a diagnosis of major depression and be alert for warning signs of suicide.

   a and b. These diagnoses fail to address the seriousness of the patient's statement.

   d. This diagnosis is more typical in patients with schizophrenia.

Analysis/Safe care/Analysis (Dx)

33. *Correct response: d*

This response communicates to the patient that the nurse is listening to her and encourages further verbalization of her pain.

   a, b, and c. These responses challenge the patient and close down further communication.

Application/Psychosocial/Implementation

34. *Correct response: c*

This response gives the nurse and the patient an opportunity to negotiate on one part of her behavior. The nurse is including the patient in the planning and assisting the patient in regulating her behavior.

   a, b, and d. None of these responses promotes the patient's self-esteem and ability to control her behavior or provides alternatives for acceptable behavior.

Application/Psychosocial/Implementation

35. *Correct response: b*
The combination of giving away one's prized possessions and abrupt, threatening changes in one's life is a known warning sign of suicide.
 a, c, and d. Losses may enhance depression, grief, and separation anxiety, but the giving away of prized possessions in conjunction with an anticipated loss signal something more serious than grief, depression, and separation anxiety.
Comprehension/Psychosocial/Analysis (Dx)

36. *Correct response: a*
Discharge planning involves specifically delineating the outpatient treatment regimen for the patient.
 b, c, and d. These plans do not address the patient's continued treatment after discharge.
Knowledge/Psychosocial/Planning

37. *Correct response: b*
In catatonic schizophrenia, the motor disturbances can consist of periods of immobility and strange posturing or periods of extreme excitability. Mutism can also occur.
 a and d. Delusions and hallucinations typically occur in paranoid schizophrenia.
 c. Disorganized behavior and incoherence are associated with disorganized schizophrenia.
Knowledge/Psychosocial/Assessment

38. *Correct response: c*
As with many illnesses, a combination of genetic, biologic, and environmental factors is thought to contribute to the cause of schizophrenia.
 a. This is an outdated theory about schizophrenia. Past family research has been deemed inconclusive because no control groups were used.
 b and d. These are areas of research, but no conclusive evidence

of causative factors has been found.
Comprehension/Physiologic/Assessment

39. *Correct response: b*
Paranoid delusional disorder involves a specific, confined delusion with no major impairment in role functioning.
 a and c. These are types of schizophrenia, a more severe disorder.
 d. Agoraphobia is an anxiety-related disorder.
Comprehension/Psychosocial/Analysis (Dx)

40. *Correct response: a*
Sometimes patients do not admit to altered perceptions. The nurse should observe how the patient functions in the milieu and look for subtle cues about how the environment is interpreted.
 b and c. These factors are less comprehensive than those listed in response "a."
 d. These assessment data would not be relevant to the question being asked.
Comprehension/Psychosocial/Analysis (Dx)

41. *Correct response: a*
Under this outcome, goal-specific behaviors that demonstrate realistic interpretation could be listed.
 b. The ability to perform self-hygiene is not necessarily impaired when a patient distorts the environment.
 c and d. These could be components of response "a."
Application/Psychosocial/Planning

42. *Correct response: c*
Firm, nonpunitive limit setting and a structured environment are the best approach to a verbally hostile patient.
 a and b. These measures are too severe, considering that the outbursts are brief and there is no escalation to physical violence.
 d. This approach would not be as useful as setting a clear limit on inappropriate behavior. However, this

could be a useful strategy in some cases.

Application/Safe care/Implementation

43. **Correct response: a**
The best approach with a withdrawn patient is to initiate brief, nondemanding activities on a one-to-one basis. This gives the nurse an opportunity to establish a trusting relationship with the patient.
   b and c. These approaches will overwhelm a severely withdrawn patient.
   d. Activities are a therapeutic approach used to help the patient reinvest into reality.

Application/Psychosocial/Implementation

44. **Correct response: b**
The best approach with delusional ideas is to avoid directly arguing with them yet at the same time present reality. It is also important to respond to the underlying message or affect. In this case, the patient is frightened, so the nurse addresses that by saying she believes he is safe here.
   a. This response would be premature. When the patient is better, it may be possible to discuss delusions as part of the illness.
   c and d. These responses place too much focus on the delusions.

Application/Safe care/Implementation

45. **Correct response: d**
Work history is not as relevant to the sexual problem as the other answers. The sexual problem can be diagnosed without knowing work history.
   a. A physical exam is necessary to determine any physical origins of the sexual problem.
   b. Certain illnesses and medications affect sexual functioning, and this information is essential to diagnosis.
   c. A sex history provides needed information about the history of the sexual problem and the adequacy of past sexual functioning.

Knowledge/Psychosocial/Assessment

46. **Correct response: a**
The diagnosis of Altered Sexuality Patterns is consistent with the patient's complaint and with the limited information presented here. Nonassertive behavior would make it difficult for her to meet her sexual needs.
   b. A specific dysfunction is identified after a sex history is taken and common causes of inhibited arousal are ruled out or identified as present in this case.
   c. This diagnosis implies that the sexual complaint is not a primary problem. It is common for health professionals to ignore or avoid directly addressing a sexual complaint because of uncomfortable feelings or lack of knowledge about sexuality.
   d. This diagnosis could be correct, because body image can be related to unsatisfactory sexual functioning. However, the sexual concern is not addressed in this diagnosis. Also, depression is a medical diagnosis, not a nursing diagnosis.

Application/Psychosocial/Analysis (Dx)

47. **Correct response: c**
At the intermediate level of the nurse's intervention, teaching about normal sexual response, clarifying sexual problems, and deciding on alternatives to resolve problems are addressed. This goal is measurable and realistic.
   a. This patient's problem does not relate to sexual orientation or pattern of sexual expression.
   b. This goal is at the advanced level of sex therapy.
   d. This intervention is less direct in addressing the problem and is focused on the past. It could, however, help the patient to clarify her sexual attitudes, which may be necessary later.

Analysis/Psychosocial/Planning

48. **Correct response: d**
Sensate focus activity helps increase sexual sensation to the extent possible.
   a. This does not address the patient's immediate concern.

b. This limits teaching to only one activity and area of stimulation to increase sexual sensation.

c. This is too general to give the patient needed guidance in maximizing sensations that remain.

Application/Health promotion/ Implementation

49. Correct response: d
The patient is being evaluated in this instance rather than her husband.

a, b, and c. All of these factors would be considered in evaluation.

Comprehension/Psychosocial/Evaluation

50. Correct response: b
By using this approach, the nurse can be sure that his or her own values are not influencing the decisions. The nurse needs to monitor planning and intervention with this patient to avoid value imposition.

a. This patient has conflicting feelings about his sexual orientation, which needs to be explored prior to setting goals of adapting to his sexual orientation.

c. This patient's depression and his sexual orientation are related. Both need to be addressed.

d. It is not necessary to modify personal values for a nurse to work with a patient. The nurse needs to acknowledge his or her own values and monitor responses to the patient to avoid value imposition.

Application/Safe care/Planning

51. Correct response: a
The patient indicates that she wants to be heterosexual and that she has lesbian feelings. Her conflict needs to be thoroughly explored so she can identify her sexual orientation.

b. Although this sexual event is significant in her development, and she will need to explore its meaning, it may or may not be therapeutic to include her parents in it at this time.

c and d. These criteria are incorrect for the same reasons. Both would be premature, because the patient has not yet explored and identified her sexual orientation.

Analysis/Psychosocial/Evaluation

52. Correct response: a
Alcohol dependence is characterized by an increase in the amount of alcohol consumed, the inability to control consumption, physical complications, and blackouts.

b and d. These are subsumed under alcohol dependence.

c. Blackouts and tolerance are not characteristic of alcohol abuse.

Analysis/Psychosocial/Analysis (Dx)

53. Correct response: b
Mr. Baker's statement that he drinks because of a nagging wife is an example of rationalization, justification for his drinking.

a, c, and d. Neither projection, sublimation, nor displacement is occurring in this situation.

Comprehension/Psychosocial/Analysis (Dx)

54. Correct response: b
The nurse's attitudes can impact on the treatment of Ms. Davis. Negative attitudes can be indirectly communicated and can damage the patient's self-esteem.

a and c. Neither of these should be the first intervention, and they should be done only when the nurse can demonstrate respect and a nonjudgmental attitude.

d. This is incorrect as the first intervention, although it may prove helpful for the nurse who lacks information about female addicts.

Application/Safe care/Planning

55. Correct response: b
Babies born to heroin-dependent women are also dependent and need to be withdrawn.

> a, c, and d. These is no evidence to support any of these claims.

Comprehension/Health promotion/Analysis (Dx)

56. Correct response: b
Abdominal injury is in fact the most common form of abuse toward pregnant women, although the others can and do occur.

Knowledge/Safe care/Assessment

57. Correct response: d
Observers are affected by dysfunction in the family system and often require help in coping with their emotional responses.
- a. Nonvictims are involved passively and can assist in resolving family difficulties.
- b. The available data do not support the assumption that victims are more traumatized.
- c. This approach supports family alienation and may not be indicated in the majority of cases.

Analysis/Psychosocial/Planning

58. Correct response: c
Difficulty with intrafamilial communication can be explored and altered in therapy where all members participate.
- a, b, and d. Although dyadic sessions with either the survivor or the abuser (or both) may be indicated to work on individual issues, private therapy is not the most expeditious way of addressing family communications.

Application/Psychosocial/Implementation

59. Correct response: d
The patient's physical and possibly (given her history) emotional well-being may be compromised.
- a. This would be a premature conclusion based on insufficient information.
- b. Frequent urinary tract infections can

indicate sexual abuse; the professional nurse incorporates new data in making evaluations.
- c. This suggests an inadequate assessment and possibly participation in the patient's denial.

Comprehension/Physiologic/Evaluation

60. Correct response: d
Socioeconomic status is not a reliable predictor of abuse in the home environment.
- a. A safe, supportive environment for abuse survivors is a valuable, necessary asset.
- b. The nurse should identify family resources available to the patient.
- c. An abuse victim's trauma can be compounded by feelings of guilt and (unreasonable) responsibility if only the abuser leaves the home environment.

Application/Safe care/Analysis (Dx)

61. Correct response: a
Psychodynamic theories identify the need to resolve conflicts associated with history of past abuse and impaired impulse control as predisposing factors for abusive behavior.
- b. Social learning theory stresses impaired learning due to dysfunctional examples.
- c. Epidemiologic factors are not considered.
- d. Environmental stress and social values issues also are not applicable.

Analysis/Psychosocial/Planning

62. Correct response: c
Persons with a diagnosis of major depression usually experience disinterest (anhedonia) and consequently lack an appetite, because food no longer tastes good.
- a, b, and d. These are all symptoms of anorexia nervosa.

Comprehension/Safe care/Assessment

63. Correct response: c
Persons with a diagnosis of major depression typically exhibit symptoms of

social isolation. The appropriate short-term goal, therefore, is group attendance.

   a and b. These are long-term goals.

   d. This is an intermediate goal that will be achieved after Mary begins to feel comfortable in the group.

Application/Psychosocial/Planning

64. *Correct response: a*

This response assists Mary in exploring and evaluating her feelings about psychiatric hospitalization.

   b. This response challenges Mary.

   c and d. These responses fail to maintain the focus on Mary's feelings.

Application/Psychosocial/Implementation

65. *Correct response: b*

Nurses need to be cognizant of counter-transference and to seek supervision or counseling to reduce its negative impact.

   a, c, and d. All of these actions would be nontherapeutic for the adolescent and her parents because they are related to the nurse's own unresolved family issues.

Analysis/Psychosocial/Assessment

66. *Correct response: a*

Susan's preoccupation with food is maintained by this interaction; therefore, it is not therapeutic.

   b, c, and d. These are all incorrect interpretations of the situation.

Analysis/Psychosocial/Evaluation

67. *Correct response: b*

A key evaluation tool for persons with a diagnosis of anorexia nervosa is weight gain.

   a, c, and d. Socialization, interest, and personal hygiene are generally not key problems.

Comprehension/Psychosocial/Evaluation

68. *Correct response: c*

The patient's statements are an example of transference—an overidealization of the nurse. Accepting these statements only reinforces this unrealistic view and prevents the patient from dealing with unresolved issues.

   a and b. It is not helpful to support beliefs and to enhance self-esteem on erroneous information.

   d. The patient's statements are unrelated to his world view in this particular situation.

Analysis/Psychosocial/Implementation

69. *Correct response: a*

Some type of behavior modification is characteristic of all milieu therapies.

   b, c, and d. These may or may not be components of a particular milieu therapy.

Knowledge/Psychosocial/Implementation

70. *Correct response: c*

The three factors considered to affect the equilibrium of a person in crisis are perception of the event, situational support, and coping skills.

   a, b, and d. These are other factors not necessarily highlighted within the crisis model.

Knowledge/Psychosocial/Assessment

71. *Correct response: b*

Shock and disbelief constitute the first stage of the grieving process. In this phase, the family is trying to realize that the loved one is really dead.

   a and d. These actions typically occur after grief is resolved.

   c. These feelings are more typical of the second phase of grieving.

Comprehension/Psychosocial/Assessment

72. *Correct response: a*

Grieving is common to all humans, because death touches everyone's life at some time. It is an important task to complete the grieving process and experience the painful feelings. If these are not experienced, psychiatric symptoms, such as agitated depression, can occur.

b, c, and d. These responses do not reflect knowledge about normal grieving.
Comprehension/Psychosocial/Analysis (Dx)

73. *Correct response: b*
Mrs. Jonas's symptoms are typical of the somatic symptoms experienced in early grieving.
   a and c. These responses fail to acknowledge that grief is manifested somatically.
   d. The somatic symptoms are a normal expression of grief.
Comprehension/Psychosocial/Analysis (Dx)

74. *Correct response: a*
Crisis intervention is based on the idea that a crisis is an upset in a steady state. The goal is to help the person return to a previous state of equilibrium.
   b, c, and d. These are not considered the primary outcome of crisis intervention, although they may occur as a side benefit.
Knowledge/Psychosocial/Evaluation

75. *Correct response: b*
A crisis persisting for more than 3 months usually indicates a more serious problem requiring more help than is given in the typical crisis intervention approach.
   a, c, and d. These analyses may or may not be true in this situation; not enough information is given about the situation.
Comprehension/Psychosocial/Analysis (Dx)

76. *Correct response: b*
The initiation phase is characterized by increased anxiety and uncertainty.
   a, c, and d. Group members are more self-reliant in these phases.
Comprehension/Psychosocial/Assessment

77. *Correct response: d*
During the initiation phase, the leader's goals should include providing directions and clarifying group purposes.

a, b, and c. Focusing on self-awareness and conflict, as well as providing minimal directions, in the beginning phase of group therapy would only increase group members' anxiety.
Comprehension/Psychosocial/Planning

78. *Correct response: b*
The use of the pronouns "our" and "we" enhances the sense of the group as a viable unit.
   a and c. This response doesn't restrict group spontaneity and it does address norms; listening is important.
   d. The purpose of group therapy is not to prevent conflict but rather to monitor conflict.
Analysis/Psychosocial/Implementation

79. *Correct response: c*
The group leader must not only observe and identify, and be cognizant of scapegoating as a common phenomenon in group therapy, but must primarily help members to deal effectively with this type of interaction.
   a, b, and d. These would be inappropriate approaches.
Application/Psychosocial/Implementation

80. *Correct response: a*
As the group progresses into the working phase, group members are to assume more responsibility for the group; the leader becomes a facilitator. Group members making statements indicating progress is a good indicator that they are becoming more active and involved.
   b, c, and d. These actions would indicate hindered group progress.
Analysis/Psychosocial/Evaluation

81. *Correct response: b*
During termination, it is very important for group members to evaluate the progress of the group and of themselves.
   a and d. These actions would fail to handle the issue of termina-

tion by denying and avoiding it, respectively.

c. This response would fail to deal with all the issues of termination (i.e., both negative and positive experiences are to be reviewed).

Comprehension/Psychosocial/Evaluation

82. *Correct response: b*

Whatever is taking place in the subgroup can and should be explored by the group in order to reduce the negative impact of subgrouping (i.e., increased group conflict and decreased group cohesiveness).

a, c, and d. These actions would not assist the group in resolving conflict.

Application/Psychosocial/Implementation

83. *Correct response: a*

Observation of the physical environment and the interactions taking place constitutes assessment.

b, c, and d. No nursing intervention, planning, or evaluation has occurred in the scenario.

Comprehension/Psychosocial/Assessment

84. *Correct response: b*

The nurse's own feelings and thoughts can have a negative impact on the therapeutic relationship. If the nurse finds that she cannot be therapeutic, she needs to refer the couple and seek supervision.

a, c, and d. These responses are inappropriate and reflect the nurse's biases.

Application/Psychosocial/Implementation

85. *Correct response: c*

The nurse has given the family specific suggestions on their interaction to be accomplished before the next visit.

a, b, and d. Neither prescribing of symptoms, reframing, nor assigning within-session tasks occurred in this scenario.

Application/Psychosocial/Implementation

86. *Correct response: d*

Instructing mother and daughter to do something fun together challenges their old patterns of interacting.

a, b, and c. These do not accurately describe the rationale for the nursing action.

Application/Psychosocial/Planning

87. *Correct response: b*

The fact that the mother and daughter did not complete the homework assignment provides further important information about the family.

a and c. Noncompliance is not considered a failure in this case.

d. The mother and daughter's return to the session may or may not be related to this intervention.

Analysis/Psychosocial/Evaluation

88. *Correct response: b*

Reframing rephrases the symptom and gives it a different meaning for the purpose of reducing family tension.

a, c, and d. In this situation, symptoms were not prescribed, assignments were not given, and feelings were not emphasized, respectively.

Application/Psychosocial/Implementation

89. *Correct response: c*

The primary purpose of family intervention is to effect behavioral change.

a, b, and d. These evaluation criteria maintain the same family behavioral patterns that led to the problem.

Application/Psychosocial/Evaluation

90. *Correct response: b*

Impaired verbal communication provides a system-oriented diagnosis.

a, c, and d. These are all more individually oriented diagnoses.

Application/Psychosocial/Analysis (Dx)

91. *Correct response: b*

The primary tasks of newlyweds are to establish themselves as a unit, to develop and maintain loyalty to that unit, to renegotiate their relationships with their family of origin, and to decide whether or not to have children.

    a, c, and d. These tasks will face the couple later in their development.

Knowledge/Psychosocial/Assessment

92. *Correct response: b*

These are classic symptoms of dystonia.

    a. The specificity of these symptoms is more suggestive of dystonia than of tension.

    c. Symptoms of pseudoparkinsonism are experienced as akinesia or generalized rigidity, drooling.

    d. Toxicity is rare and typically develops over the course of days; symptoms are characterized by high fever, muscular rigidity, tremors, and hyperkalemia.

Application/Safe care/Analysis (Dx)

93. *Correct response: a*

The converse is also true; lower-potency drugs tend to produce less dystonic episodes.

    b. Dystonia occurs in 10% of EPS presentations, so it is not that common; the current trend is not to administer antiparkinsonian drugs routinely because they may not be necessary.

    c. The emergence of dystonia has no bearing on the effectiveness of the medication.

    d. Stelazine 2 mg t.i.d. is not a high dose; toxic side effects are rare, and when they do occur they are not limited to the stabilization period.

Comprehension/Physiologic/Analysis (Dx)

94. *Correct response: c*

Patients report feeling frightened with the abrupt emergence of a dystonic reaction.

    a, b, and d. Dystonia tends to incite fearful emotions that relate to feeling out of control of one's body and being unclear about the cause of the acute symptoms coupled with intense physical manifestations.

Comprehension/Psychosocial/Planning

95. *Correct response: c*

Immediate injection (IM or IV) of antiparkinsonian medication will effect rapid relief of dystonia.

    a. Obtaining a blood sample would not be indicated; toxicity is not the issue.

    b. This is not necessary because the antiparkinsonian medication will attenuate these symptoms.

    d. Mr. Joad's symptoms are clearly physiologic and require immediate pharmacologic intervention.

Application/Safe care/Implementation

96. *Correct response: b*

An increase in the antipsychotic medication would probably result in an increase in EPS.

    a, c, and d. All of these actions would appropriately manage the side effects of the antipsychotic medication.

Comprehension/Safe care/Evaluation

Index

Page numbers followed by *d* indicate displays; page numbers followed by *f* indicate figures; page numbers followed by *t* indicate tabular material.

Psychotic disorders. *See also* Schizophrenic
   disorders
   definition of, 75
Psychotic responses, in schizophrenia, 77

Q

Questions, open-ended, therapeutic communication and, 6

R

Rational-emotive therapy, 22
Rationalization, anxiety and, 36
Reaction formation, anxiety and, 36
Receiver, in therapeutic communication, 5
Recognition-seeker, 179
Reflecting, therapeutic communication and,
   7
Relaxation techniques, 20
   stress reduction and, 33
Repression, anxiety and, 36
Residual schizophrenia, 78–79
Resolution phase of sexual response, 94
Restating, therapeutic communication and,
   6
Restlessness, tricyclic antidepressants and,
   215
Rifampicin, drug interactions of, 224
Role(s)
   in group, 178–179
   therapeutic communication and, 6

S

Satisfaction drive, 20
Scapegoating, 192
Schismatic situation, 192
Schizophrenic disorders, 75–83
   basic concepts of, 75–76
   catatonic, 78
   in childhood and adolescence, 148
   definition of, 75
   disorganized, 78
   etiology of, 76–77
   general characteristics of, 76
   nursing process and, 79–83
      assessment and, 79–80
      evaluation and, 82–83
      nursing diagnoses and, 80
      planning and implementation and,
         80–82, 81d
   paranoid, 78
   psychosocial implications of, 77–78

residual, 78–79
   undifferentiated, 78
Secondary prevention, 3
Security drive, 20
Sedation
   antipsychotic drugs and, 208
   tricyclic antidepressants and, 215
Sedative-hypnotic drugs, 221–225
   abuse of, 115–118
   administration of, 223
   adverse side effects of, 224
   contraindications to, 223
   drug interactions of, 224–225
   general considerations with, 222
   indications for, 221–222
   mechanisms of action of, 222
   patient education and, nursing implica-
      tions in, 224
   selection of, 222–223
   sexual dysfunction due to, 100
Seizures
   antipsychotic drugs and, 208
   tricyclic antidepressants and, 216
Self, offering, therapeutic communication
   and, 6
Self-confessor, 179
Self-help groups, 181
Seligman's theory, affective disorders and,
   61
Sender, in therapeutic communication, 5
Sexual abuse, 131. *See also* Family violence
Sexual acting-out, 97
Sexual alterations, 91–106
   gender identity and, 96–97
   mild, 94–95
   moderate, 95
   nursing process in, 101–106
      analysis and nursing diagnoses and,
         102
      assessment and, 101–102
      evaluation and, 106
      planning and implementation and,
         102–105
   severe, 95
   sexual addictions and, 101
   sexual behavior and, 97–98
   sexual dysfunction and, 98–101
      due to drugs and surgery, 100–101
      painful, 99–100
   sexual orientation and, 97
   tricyclic antidepressants and, 216
Sexuality. *See also* Sexual alterations
   characteristic patterns of expression or ori-
      entation and, 95–96